50% OFF Online HESI A2 Prep Course!

Dear Customer,

We consider it an honor and a privilege that you chose our HESI A2 Study Guide. As a way of showing our appreciation and to help us better serve you, we have partnered with Mometrix Test Preparation to offer **50% off their online HESI A2 Prep Course.** Many HESI A2 courses are needlessly expensive and don't deliver enough value. With their course, you get access to the best HESI A2 prep material, and you only pay half price.

Mometrix has structured their online course to perfectly complement your printed study guide. The HESI A2 Prep Course contains **over 100 lessons** that cover all the most important topics, **90+ video reviews** that explain difficult concepts, **over 2,000 practice questions** to ensure you feel prepared, and **digital flashcards**, so you can fit some studying in while you're on the go.

Online HESI A2 Prep Course

Topics Covered:

- Reading
  - o Key Ideas and Details
  - o Craft and Structure
  - o Integration of Knowledge & Ideas
- English & Language Usage
  - o Conventions of Standard English
  - o Knowledge of Language
  - o Vocabulary Acquisition
- Science
  - o Human Anatomy & Physiology
  - o Life & Physical Sciences
  - o Scientific Reasoning
- Math
  - o Numbers & Algebra
  - o Measurement & Data

Course Features:

- HESI A2 Study Guide
  - o Get content that complements our best-selling study guide.
- 7 Full-Length Practice Tests
  - o With over 2,000 practice questions, you can test yourself again and again.
- Mobile Friendly
  - o If you need to study on-the-go, the course is easily accessible from your mobile device.
- HESI A2 Flashcards
  - o The course includes a flashcard mode consisting of over 300 content cards to help you study.

To receive this discount, simply head to their website: mometrix.com/university/hesi or simply scan this QR code with your smartphone. At the checkout page, enter the discount code: **APEXHESI50**

If you have any questions or concerns, please don't hesitate to contact Mometrix at universityhelp@mometrix.com.

SCAN HERE

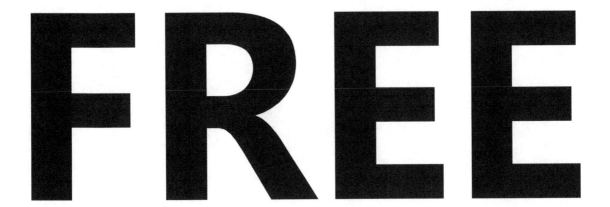

Free Study Tips DVD

In addition to the tips and content in this guide, we have created a FREE DVD with helpful study tips to further assist your exam preparation. **This FREE Study Tips DVD provides you with top-notch tips to conquer your exam and reach your goals.**

Our simple request in exchange for the strategy-packed DVD is that you email us your feedback about our study guide. We would love to hear what you thought about the guide, and we welcome any and all feedback—positive, negative, or neutral. It is our #1 goal to provide you with top quality products and customer service.

To receive your **FREE Study Tips DVD**, email freedvd@apexprep.com. Please put "FREE DVD" in the subject line and put the following in the email:

   a. The name of the study guide you purchased.

   b. Your rating of the study guide on a scale of 1-5, with 5 being the highest score.

   c. Any thoughts or feedback about your study guide.

   d. Your first and last name and your mailing address, so we know where to send your free DVD!

Thank you!

HESI A2 Study Guide 2021-2022
HESI Admission Assessment Exam Review with Practice Test Questions [Updated for New Outline]

Matthew Lanni

Written and edited by APEX Publishing.

ISBN 13: 9781637757352
ISBN 10: 1637757352

APEX Publishing is not connected with or endorsed by any official testing organization. APEX Publishing creates and publishes unofficial educational products. All test and organization names are trademarks of their respective owners.

The material in this publication is included for utilitarian purposes only and does not constitute an endorsement by APEX Publishing of any particular point of view.

For additional information or for bulk orders, contact info@apexprep.com.

Table of Contents

Test Taking Strategies

1. Reading the Whole Question

A popular assumption in Western culture is the idea that we don't have enough time for anything. We speed while driving to work, we want to read an assignment for class as quickly as possible, or we want the line in the supermarket to dwindle faster. However, speeding through such events robs us from being able to thoroughly appreciate and understand what's happening around us. While taking a timed test, the feeling one might have while reading a question is to find the correct answer as quickly as possible. Although pace is important, don't let it deter you from reading the whole question. Test writers know how to subtly change a test question toward the end in various ways, such as adding a negative or changing focus. If the question has a passage, carefully read the whole passage as well before moving on to the questions. This will help you process the information in the passage rather than worrying about the questions you've just read and where to find them. A thorough understanding of the passage or question is an important way for test takers to be able to succeed on an exam.

2. Examining Every Answer Choice

Let's say we're at the market buying apples. The first apple we see on top of the heap may *look* like the best apple, but if we turn it over we can see bruising on the skin. We must examine several apples before deciding which apple is the best. Finding the correct answer choice is like finding the best apple. Although it's tempting to choose an answer that seems correct at first without reading the others, it's important to read each answer choice thoroughly before making a final decision on the answer. The aim of a test writer might be to get as close as possible to the correct answer, so watch out for subtle words that may indicate an answer is incorrect. Once the correct answer choice is selected, read the question again and the answer in response to make sure all your bases are covered.

3. Eliminating Wrong Answer Choices

Sometimes we become paralyzed when we are confronted with too many choices. Which frozen yogurt flavor is the tastiest? Which pair of shoes look the best with this outfit? What type of car will fill my needs as a consumer? If you are unsure of which answer would be the best to choose, it may help to use process of elimination. We use "filtering" all the time on sites such as eBay® or Craigslist® to eliminate the ads that are not right for us. We can do the same thing on an exam. Process of elimination is crossing out the answer choices we know for sure are wrong and leaving the ones that might be correct. It may help to cover up the incorrect answer choice. Covering incorrect choices is a psychological act that alleviates stress due to the brain being exposed to a smaller amount of information. Choosing between two answer choices is much easier than choosing between all of them, and you have a better chance of selecting the correct answer if you have less to focus on.

4. Sticking to the World of the Question

When we are attempting to answer questions, our minds will often wander away from the question and what it is asking. We begin to see answer choices that are true in the real world instead of true in the world of the question. It may be helpful to think of each test question as its own little world. This world may be different from ours. This world may know as a truth that the chicken came before the egg or may assert that two plus two equals five. Remember that, no matter what hypothetical nonsense may be in the question, assume it to be true. If the question states that the chicken came before the egg, then choose your answer based on that truth. Sticking to the world of the question means placing all of our biases and assumptions aside and relying on the question to guide us to the correct answer. If we are simply looking for answers that are correct based on our own judgment, then we may choose incorrectly. Remember an answer that is true does not necessarily answer the question.

5. Key Words

If you come across a complex test question that you have to read over and over again, try pulling out some key words from the question in order to understand what exactly it is asking. Key words may be words that surround the question, such as *main idea, analogous, parallel, resembles, structured,* or *defines*. The question may be asking for the main idea, or it may be asking you to define something. Deconstructing the sentence may also be helpful in making the question simpler before trying to answer it. This means taking the sentence apart and obtaining meaning in pieces, or separating the question from the foundation of the question. For example, let's look at this question:

> Given the author's description of the content of paleontology in the first paragraph, which of the following is most parallel to what it taught?

The question asks which one of the answers most *parallels* the following information: The *description* of paleontology in the first paragraph. The first step would be to see *how* paleontology is described in the first paragraph. Then, we would find an answer choice that parallels that description. The question seems complex at first, but after we deconstruct it, the answer becomes much more attainable.

6. Subtle Negatives

Negative words in question stems will be words such as *not, but, neither,* or *except*. Test writers often use these words in order to trick unsuspecting test takers into selecting the wrong answer—or, at least, to test their reading comprehension of the question. Many exams will feature the negative words in all caps (*which of the following is NOT an example*), but some questions will add the negative word seamlessly into the sentence. The following is an example of a subtle negative used in a question stem:

> According to the passage, which of the following is *not* considered to be an example of paleontology?

If we rush through the exam, we might skip that tiny word, *not*, inside the question, and choose an answer that is opposite of the correct choice. Again, it's important to read the question fully, and double check for any words that may negate the statement in any way.

7. Spotting the Hedges

The word "hedging" refers to language that remains vague or avoids absolute terminology. Absolute terminology consists of words like *always, never, all, every, just, only, none,* and *must*. Hedging refers to words like *seem, tend, might, most, some, sometimes, perhaps, possibly, probability,* and *often*. In some cases, we want to choose answer choices that use hedging and avoid answer choices that use absolute terminology. It's important to pay attention to what subject you are on and adjust your response accordingly.

8. Restating to Understand

Every now and then we come across questions that we don't understand. The language may be too complex, or the question is structured in a way that is meant to confuse the test taker. When you come across a question like this, it may be worth your time to rewrite or restate the question in your own words in order to understand it better. For example, let's look at the following complicated question:

> Which of the following words, if substituted for the word *parochial* in the first paragraph, would LEAST change the meaning of the sentence?

Let's restate the question in order to understand it better. We know that they want the word *parochial* replaced. We also know that this new word would "least" or "not" change the meaning of the sentence. Now let's try the sentence again:

> Which word could we replace with *parochial,* and it would not change the meaning?

Restating it this way, we see that the question is asking for a synonym. Now, let's restate the question so we can answer it better:

> Which word is a synonym for the word *parochial?*

Before we even look at the answer choices, we have a simpler, restated version of a complicated question.

9. Predicting the Answer

After you read the question, try predicting the answer *before* reading the answer choices. By formulating an answer in your mind, you will be less likely to be distracted by any wrong answer choices. Using predictions will also help you feel more confident in the answer choice you select. Once you've chosen your answer, go back and reread the question and answer choices to make sure you have the best fit. If you have no idea what the answer may be for a particular question, forego using this strategy.

10. Avoiding Patterns

One popular myth in grade school relating to standardized testing is that test writers will often put multiple-choice answers in patterns. A runoff example of this kind of thinking is that the most common answer choice is "C," with "B" following close behind. Or, some will advocate certain made-up word patterns that simply do not exist. Test writers do not arrange their correct answer choices in any kind of pattern; their choices are randomized. There may even be times where the correct answer choice will be the same letter for two or three questions in a row, but we have no way of knowing when or if this might happen. Instead of trying to figure out what choice the test writer probably set as being correct, focus on what the *best answer choice* would be out of the answers you are presented with. Use the tips above, general knowledge, and reading comprehension skills in order to best answer the question, rather than looking for patterns that do not exist.

FREE DVD OFFER

Achieving a high score on your exam depends not only on understanding the content, but also on understanding how to apply your knowledge and your command of test taking strategies. **Because your success is our primary goal, we offer a FREE Study Tips DVD, which provides top-notch test taking strategies to help you optimize your testing experience.**

Our simple request in exchange for the strategy-packed DVD is that you email us your feedback about our study guide.

To receive your **FREE Study Tips DVD**, email freedvd@apexprep.com. Please put "FREE DVD" in the subject line and put the following in the email:

    a. The name of the study guide you purchased.

    b. Your rating of the study guide on a scale of 1-5, with 5 being the highest score.

    c. Any thoughts or feedback about your study guide.

    d. Your first and last name and your mailing address, so we know where to send your free DVD!

Introduction to the HESI Admission Assessment Exam

Function of the Test

The Health Education Systems, Inc. Admission Assessment Exam, also called the HESI A2, is an entrance exam used by nursing programs to help determine a candidate's admission status. Most test takers are finishing up high school or are recent high school graduates seeking admission to a nursing program or other post-secondary health program. Each nursing program can set their own minimum passing scores that candidates must achieve to be granted admission to the program. Additionally, although there are ten potential sections or subtests of the HESI A2 (eight of which are academic subjects), nursing programs can select just a subset of these offerings, meaning that test takers may not need scores in all eight academic categories to be considered for admission. Test takers should check with the schools they are interested in applying to for an accurate list of the required HESI A2 section scores. The subtests that are not academic in nature include a learning style test and a personality test.

Test Administration

Applicants usually take the HESI A2 at the institution where they intend to apply. The test is administered online and while most schools that include the exam as part of their admissions process offer the exam at various times on-site, some Prometric test centers also offer administration of the HESI A2. Because many of the specifics of the exam administration are left to the discretion of each nursing program, the testing experience will vary at different testing institutions. For example, the cost for the exam, the available dates and times of administration, and the required sections are determined by each school. Additionally, some programs may allow candidates to retake the test or combine the highest scores achieved on the various subtests over multiple administrations to obtain the best composite scores, while other programs may prohibit retesting or may only accept scores obtained from one coherent session. Test takers are encouraged to inquire about all the testing specifics at each institution on their prospective application list. Accommodations for documented disabilities are usually permitted, though test takers should contact nursing programs directly to arrange for any necessary accommodations.

Test Format

The HESI A2 contains four major sections: English Language, Math, Science, and a Personality Profile. The English Language section consists of three 55-question sections: Reading Comprehension, Vocabulary & General Knowledge, and Grammar. The Math section also contains 55 questions. The Science section consists of four 30-question tests: Biology, Chemistry, Anatomy & Physiology, and Physics. The Personality Profile consists of a 15-question Personality Profile and a 14-question Learning Style assessment.

Again, because each school or testing center can establish their own testing schedule and required sections, universal set time limits do not exist for the HESI A2. With that said, typically, test takers are allotted 5.25 hours total in cases where all ten sections are administered.

The following chart summarizes the sections on the HESI A2:

Section	Questions
English- Reading Comprehension	55
English- Vocabulary & Knowledge	55
English- Grammar	55
Mathematics	55
Science- Biology	30
Science- Chemistry	30
Science- Anatomy & Physiology	30
Science- Physics	30
Personality Profile	14
Learning Style	15

Scoring

After a candidate completes the exam, he or she will receive a detailed score report as will the nursing program that administered the exam. The score report contains an explanation of the scoring process and scores for each of the subtests attempted. Scores are typically presented as a percentage of questions answered correctly; there is no penalty for incorrect answers, so test takers should not leave questions blank. As mentioned, each nursing program determines the minimum passing score for prospective students; there is no set passing score for the HESI A2. With that said, many RN programs establish a minimum score of 75%.

Study Prep Plan Template for the HESI Admission Assessment Exam

1 **Breathe**

Reducing stress is key when preparing for your test.

2 **Build**

Create a study plan to help you stay on track.

3 **Begin**

Stick with your study plan. You've got this!

1 Week Study Plan

Day 1	Day 2	Day 3	Day 4	Day 5	Day 6	Day 7
						Take your exam!

2 Week Study Plan

Day 1	Day 2	Day 3	Day 4	Day 5	Day 6	Day 7

Day 8	Day 9	Day 10	Day 11	Day 12	Day 13	Day 14
						Take your exam!

30 Day Study Plan

Day 1	Day 2	Day 3	Day 4	Day 5	Day 6	Day 7

Day 8	Day 9	Day 10	Day 11	Day 12	Day 13	Day 14

Day 15	Day 16	Day 17	Day 18	Day 19	Day 20	Day 21

Day 22	Day 23	Day 24	Day 25	Day 26	Day 27	Day 28

Day 29	Day 30
	Take your exam!

Math

Basic Operations with Whole Numbers

Addition is the combining of two numbers to find the total. The numbers being added together are the **addends**, and the resulting answer is the **sum**. Addition problems can be completed using a variety of strategies including number lines, base-10 blocks, place value, and concrete models. When adding multi-digit numbers, the numbers must be lined up by place value vertically. The problem $138 + 47$ demonstrating this type of addition involving carrying is shown below:

$$\begin{array}{r} 1\ 3\,^1 8 \\ +\quad 4\ 7 \\ \hline 1\ 8\ 5 \end{array}$$

The addition of the ones column $8 + 7 = 15$, so the 5 is written beneath the ones column, and the 1 is carried over to be added to the tens column. The remaining columns are added down to provide the solution.

When adding a negative number to a positive number, the problem becomes a subtraction problem. Adding 10 and -2 becomes:

$$10 + (-2) = 10 - 2 = 8$$

When adding two negative numbers, complete the addition as usual, but the resulting total is negative,

$$-15 + (-6) = -21$$

Subtraction involves taking away or removing an amount from a number to find the difference of the two values. Addition and subtraction are related because they are inverse operations. For example, the addition problem $7 + 2 = 9$ can be changed into a subtraction problem:

$$9 - 2 = 7$$

Subtraction problems also can be solved using some of the same methods as addition including number lines and concrete models. Subtracting multi-digit numbers is slightly more complicated because they can involve **borrowing**. An example of a subtraction problem $263 - 56$ with borrowing is shown below:

$$\begin{array}{r} 2\,^5 6\,^1 3 \\ -\quad 5\ 6 \\ \hline 2\ 0\ 7 \end{array}$$

In the ones column, 6 cannot be subtracted from 3; therefore, 1 is borrowed from the tens column making the ones column on the top row 13 instead of 3. The 6 in the tens column becomes 5 instead of 6. The rest of the subtraction is carried out accordingly.

When a negative number is subtracted, it creates a double negative, $13 - (-6)$. This changes the sign to a positive,

$$13 + 6 = 19$$

Multiplication is basically a short cut to repeated addition. For example, 4×5 can be thought of as adding the number 4 a total of 5 times: $4 + 4 + 4 + 4 + 4$. Both of these techniques yield the equivalent answer, 20. Another strategy for completing multiplication problems is to imagine sets of items being added together. One method to accomplish this is through the use of arrays. The following array represents 5 × 3.

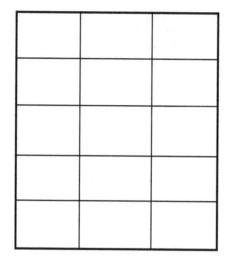

Other methods to complete multiplication problems include area models, partial products, and long multiplication like the example that follows:

```
    23
  × 14
```

```
   2¹3
  × 1 4
    9 2
```

The right column is multiplied first. In this case, 3 × 4 = 12 so the 2 is written below the right column, and the 1 is carried. Next, the 4 in the right column is multiplied by the 2 in the left column, and the 1 that was carried in the previous step is added:

$$(4 \times 2) + 1 = 9$$

The result is placed to the left of the 2.

```
    2¹3
  × 1 4
    9 2
      0
```

A 0 or blank space must be used for a placeholder before completing the next step of multiplication.

```
    2 3
  × 1 4
    9 2
  2 3 0
```

The next line of multiplication starts with the 1 in the left column. It is multiplied starting on the right by 3 and then by 2, with the results written below the appropriate columns as shown.

```
    2 3
  × 1 4
    9 2
  2¹3 0
  3 2 2
```

The two lines of multiplication are added together to achieve the final product of 322.

When multiplying negative and nonnegative numbers, if the signs are the same, then the answer is positive. If the signs are different, then the answer is negative. These same rules apply to division as well.

Like addition and subtraction, multiplication and division are inverse operations. Division splits an amount or number into equal groups or parts. For example, $14 \div 2 = 7$ because 14 can be separated into 2 equal groups of 7. In the previous example, 14 is the **dividend**, 2 is the **divisor**, and 7 is the **quotient**, which is the term for the solution to a division problem. Division problems can be solved using arrays, area models, or equal groups of concrete objects. Division of multi-digit numbers can also be completed using long division, for example, $348 \div 6$.

```
    58
 6│348
   30↓
   ──
    48
    48
   ──
     0
```

First, set up the problem. Start by dividing the first number on the left of the dividend, 3, by the divisor of 6. 3 is not divisible by 6, so the next number to the left in the dividend (the 3) comes into play. This means that 34 must be divided by 6. 6 will divide into 34 a total of 5 times, so the 5 goes above the 4.

6 multiplied by 5 equals 30, so write that below the 34. Then, subtract 30 from 34. This leaves 4. The next number to the right in the dividend must be dropped down to make 48. 48 is evenly divisible by 6, so put the quotient of that division, 8, on the top next to the 5.

The final solution is 58.

Operations follow certain properties and rules. Addition and multiplication follow the **commutative property**. This means that the numbers can be added or multiplied in any order, and the result will be the same. For example, $6 \times 3 = 18$ and $3 \times 6 = 18$. Subtraction and division are not commutative. Addition and multiplication are also associative. The **associative property** means that the grouping of numbers with parentheses does not change the answer to the problem. For example,

$$(7 + 8) + 5 = 20 \text{ and } (7 + 5) + 8 = 20$$

Another property that impacts operations is the distributive property. The **distributive property** states that when a sum or difference inside the parentheses is multiplied by a number, it is the same as multiplying both the numbers inside the parentheses by the outside number and adding or subtracting the results. For example:

$$8 \times (4 + 3) = 8 \times 7 = 56$$

and

$$8 \times 4 + 8 \times 3 = 32 + 24 = 56$$

When using operations and their properties, it is also important to remember the rule for the order of operations. When evaluating an expression, any operations inside grouping symbols must be completed first. Next, any numbers with exponents are simplified. Then, the multiplication and division portions of the expression can be evaluated. Addition and subtraction are to be completed last. A helpful mnemonic to remember these steps is *Please Excuse My Dear Aunt Sally* or **PEMDAS**. The following expression needs to be completed using the order of operations.

$$(5 - 3) \times 6 + 8$$

The numbers inside the parentheses need to be evaluated first. This gives $2 \times 6 + 8$. Next, the multiplication must be completed, $12 + 8$. Last, the addition is completed to provide a solution:

$$12 + 8 = 20$$

Decimals

Operations can be performed on rational numbers in decimal form. In this case, it is important to keep track of place value. To add decimals, make sure the decimal places are in alignment and add vertically. If the numbers do not line up because there are extra or missing place values in one of the numbers, then zeros may be used as placeholders. For example, $0.123 + 0.23$ becomes:

$$
\begin{array}{r}
0.123 \\
+ \, 0.230 \\
\hline
0.353
\end{array}
$$

Subtraction is done the same way. Multiplication and division are more complicated. To multiply two decimals, place one on top of the other as in a regular multiplication process and do not worry about lining up the decimal points. Then, multiply as with whole numbers, ignoring the decimals. Finally, in the solution, insert the decimal point as many places to the left as there are total digits to the right of the decimal in the original problem. Here is an example of decimal multiplication:

$$
\begin{array}{rl}
0.67 & \text{2 decimal places} \\
\times \, 0.4 & \text{1 decimal place} \\
\hline
0.268 & \text{3 decimal places}
\end{array}
$$

The answer to 0.67 times 0.4 is 0.268, and because there are three decimal values in the problem, the decimal point is positioned three units to the left in the answer.

The decimal point plays an integral role throughout the whole problem when dividing with decimals. First, set up the problem in a long division format. If the divisor is not an integer, move the decimal to the right as many units as needed to make it an integer. The decimal in the dividend must be moved to the right the same number of places to maintain equality. Then, complete division normally.

Here is an example of long division with decimals:

$$12.72 \div 0.06$$

$$= \quad 0.06\overline{)12.72}$$

$$= \quad \begin{array}{r} 212 \\ 6\overline{)1272} \\ \underline{12}\downarrow \\ 07 \\ \underline{6}\downarrow \\ 12 \end{array}$$

The decimal point in 0.06 needed to move two units to the right to turn it into an integer (6), so it also needed to move two units to the right in 12.72 to make it 1,272. The result of the division is 212, and remember that a division problem can always be checked by multiplying the answer by the divisor to see if the result is equal to the dividend.

Fractions

A **rational number** is a number that can be written in the form $\frac{a}{b}$, where a and b are integers, and b is not equal to zero. In other words, rational numbers can be written in a fraction form. The value a is the **numerator,** and b is the **denominator**. If the numerator is equal to zero, the entire fraction is equal to zero. Non-negative fractions can be less than 1, equal to 1, or greater than 1. Fractions are less than 1 if the numerator is smaller (less than) than the denominator. For example, $\frac{3}{4}$ is less than 1. A fraction is equal to 1 if the numerator is equal to the denominator. For instance, $\frac{4}{4}$ is equal to 1. Finally, a fraction is greater than 1 if the numerator is greater than the denominator: the fraction $\frac{11}{4}$ is greater than 1. When the numerator is greater than the denominator, the fraction is called an **improper fraction**. An improper fraction can be converted to a **mixed number**, a combination of both a whole number and a fraction. To convert an improper fraction to a mixed number, divide the numerator by the denominator. Write down the whole number portion, and then write any remainder over the original denominator. For example, $\frac{11}{4}$ is equivalent to $2\frac{3}{4}$. Conversely, a mixed number can be converted to an improper fraction by multiplying the denominator times the whole number and adding that result to the numerator.

Adding and Subtracting Fractions

If a rational number is in fraction form, performing addition, subtraction, multiplication, and division is more complicated than when working with integers. First, consider addition. To add two fractions having the same denominator, add the numerators and then reduce the fraction. When an answer is a fraction, it should always be in lowest terms. **Lowest terms** means that every common factor between the numerator and denominator is divided out. For example:

$$\frac{2}{8} + \frac{4}{8} = \frac{6}{8} = \frac{6 \div 2}{8 \div 2} = \frac{3}{4}$$

Both the numerator and denominator of $\frac{6}{8}$ have a common factor of 2, so 2 is divided out of each value to put the fraction in lowest terms. If denominators are different in an addition problem, the fractions must be converted to have common denominators. The **least common denominator (LCD)** of all the given denominators must be found, and this value is equal to the **least common multiple (LCM)** of the denominators. This non-zero value is the smallest number that is a multiple of both denominators. Then, rewrite each original fraction as an equivalent fraction using the new denominator. Once in this form, apply the process of adding with like denominators. For example, consider $\frac{1}{3} + \frac{4}{9}$. The LCD is 9 because it is the smallest multiple of both 3 and 9. The fraction $\frac{1}{3}$ must be rewritten with 9 as its denominator. Therefore, multiply both the numerator and denominator by 3. Multiplying by $\frac{3}{3}$ is the same as multiplying by 1, which does not change the value of the fraction. Therefore, an equivalent fraction is $\frac{3}{9}$, and $\frac{1}{3} + \frac{4}{9} = \frac{3}{9} + \frac{4}{9} = \frac{7}{9}$, which is in lowest terms. Subtraction is performed in a similar manner; once the denominators are equal, the numerators are then subtracted.

Multiplying and Dividing Fractions

Common denominators are not used in multiplication and division. To multiply two fractions, multiply the numerators together and the denominators together. Then, write the result in lowest terms. For example:

$$\frac{2}{3} \times \frac{9}{4} = \frac{18}{12} = \frac{3}{2}$$

Alternatively, the fractions could be factored first to cancel out any common factors before performing the multiplication. For example:

$$\frac{2}{3} \times \frac{9}{4} = \frac{2}{3} \times \frac{3 \times 3}{2 \times 2} = \frac{3}{2}$$

This second approach is helpful when working with larger numbers, as common factors might not be obvious.

Multiplication and division of fractions are related because the division of two fractions is changed into a multiplication problem. Division of a fraction is equivalent to multiplication of the **reciprocal** of the second fraction, so that second fraction must be inverted, or "flipped," to be in reciprocal form. For example:

$$\frac{11}{15} \div \frac{3}{5}$$

$$\frac{11}{15} \times \frac{5}{3} = \frac{55}{45} = \frac{11}{9}$$

The fraction $\frac{5}{3}$ is the reciprocal of $\frac{3}{5}$. It is possible to multiply and divide numbers containing a mix of integers and fractions. In this case, convert the integer to a fraction by placing it over a denominator of 1. For example, a division problem involving an integer and a fraction is:

$$3 \div \frac{1}{2} = \frac{3}{1} \times \frac{2}{1} = \frac{6}{1} = 6$$

Changing Fractions to Decimals

Fractions can be converted to decimals. With a calculator, a fraction is converted to a decimal by dividing the numerator by the denominator. For example:

$$\frac{2}{5} = 2 \div 5 = 0.4$$

Sometimes, rounding might be necessary. Consider:

$$\frac{2}{7} = 2 \div 7 = 0.28571429$$

This decimal could be rounded for ease of use, and if it needed to be rounded to the nearest thousandth, the result would be 0.286. If a calculator is not available, a fraction can be converted to a decimal manually. First, find a number that, when multiplied by the denominator, has a value equal to 10, 100, 1,000, etc. Then, multiply both the numerator and denominator times that number. The decimal form of the fraction is equal to the new numerator with a decimal point placed as many place values to the left as there are zeros in the denominator. For example, to convert $\frac{3}{5}$ to a decimal, multiply both the numerator and denominator times 2, which results in $\frac{6}{10}$. The decimal is equal to 0.6 because there is one zero in the denominator, and so the decimal place in the numerator is moved one unit to the left.

In the case where rounding would be necessary while working without a calculator, an approximation must be found. A number close to 10, 100, 1,000, etc. can be used. For example, to convert $\frac{1}{3}$ to a decimal, the numerator and denominator can be multiplied by 33 to turn the denominator into approximately 100, which makes for an easier conversion to the equivalent decimal. This process results in $\frac{33}{99}$ and an approximate decimal of 0.33. Once in decimal form, the number can be converted to a percentage. To do so, the decimal number is multiplied by 100 and then a percent sign is placed after the number. For example, 0.614 is equal to 61.4%. In other words, the decimal place is moved two units to the right and the percentage symbol is then added.

Ratios and Proportions

Fractions appear in everyday situations, and in many scenarios, they appear in the real-world as ratios and in proportions. A **ratio** is formed when two different quantities are compared. For example, in a group of 50 people, if there are 33 females and 17 males, the ratio of females to males is 33 to 17. This expression can be written in the fraction form as $\frac{33}{50}$, where the denominator is the sum of females and males, or by using the ratio symbol, 33:17. The order of the number matters when forming ratios. In the same setting, the ratio of males to females is 17 to 33, which is equivalent to $\frac{17}{50}$ or 17:33.

A **proportion** is an equation involving two ratios. The equation:

$$\frac{a}{b} = \frac{c}{d}$$

or

$$a : b = c : d$$

is a proportion, for real numbers a, b, c, and d. Usually, in one ratio, one of the quantities is unknown, and cross-multiplication is used to solve for the unknown. Consider:

$$\frac{1}{4} = \frac{x}{5}$$

To solve for x, cross-multiply to obtain $5 = 4x$. Divide each side by 4 to obtain the solution:

$$x = \frac{5}{4}$$

It is also true that percentages are ratios in which the second term is 100 minus the first term. For example, 65% is 65:35 or $\frac{65}{100}$. Therefore, when working with percentages, one is also working with ratios.

Real-world problems frequently involve proportions. For example, consider the following problem: If 2 out of 50 pizzas are usually delivered late from a local Italian restaurant, how many would be late out of 235 orders? The following proportion would be solved with x as the unknown quantity of late pizzas:

$$\frac{2}{50} = \frac{x}{235}$$

Cross multiplying results in $470 = 50x$. Divide both sides by 50 to obtain $x = \frac{470}{50}$, which in lowest terms is equal to $\frac{47}{5}$. In decimal form, this improper fraction is equal to 9.4. Because it does not make sense to answer this question with decimals (portions of pizzas do not get delivered) the answer must be rounded. Traditional rounding rules would say that 9 pizzas would be expected to be delivered late. However, to be safe, rounding up to 10 pizzas out of 235 would probably make more sense.

Recall that a ratio is the comparison of two different quantities. Comparing 2 apples to 3 oranges results in the ratio 2:3, which can be expressed as the fraction $\frac{2}{3}$. Many real-world problems involve ratios. Often, problems with ratios involve proportions, as when two ratios are set equal to find the missing amount. However, some problems involve deciphering single ratios. For example, consider an amusement park that sold 345 tickets last Saturday. If 145 tickets were sold to adults and the rest of the tickets were sold to children, what would the ratio of the number of adult tickets to children's tickets be? A common mistake would be to say the ratio is 145:345. However, 345 is the total number of tickets sold, not the number of children's tickets. There were:

$$345 - 145 = 200$$

tickets sold to children. The correct ratio of adult to children's tickets is 145:200. As a fraction, this expression is written as $\frac{145}{345}$, which can be reduced to $\frac{29}{69}$.

Rate of change problems involve calculating a ratio of a quantity per some unit of measurement. Usually the unit of measurement is time. For example, meters per second is a common rate of change. To calculate this measurement, find the amount traveled in meters and divide by total time traveled. The result is the average speed over the entire time interval. Another common rate of change used in the real world is miles per hour. Consider the following problem that involves calculating an average rate of change in temperature. Last Saturday, the temperature at 1:00 a.m. was 34 degrees Fahrenheit, and at noon, the temperature had increased to 75 degrees Fahrenheit. What was the average rate of change over that time interval? The average rate of change is calculated by finding the change in temperature and dividing by the total hours elapsed. Therefore, the rate of change was equal to:

$$\frac{75 - 34}{12 - 1} = \frac{41}{11} \text{ degrees per hour}$$

This quantity rounded to two decimal places is equal to 3.73 degrees per hour.

Percentages

As discussed previously, percentages are defined to be parts per one hundred. To convert a decimal to a percentage, the decimal point is moved two units to the right and the percent sign is placed after the number. Percentages appear in many scenarios in the real world. It is important to make sure the statement containing the percentage is translated to a correct mathematical expression. Be aware that it is extremely common to make a mistake when working with percentages within word problems.

An example of a word problem containing a percentage is the following: 35% of people speed when driving to work. In a group of 5,600 commuters, how many would be expected to speed on the way to their place of employment? The answer to this problem is found by finding 35% of 5,600. To do this, first, change the percentage to the decimal 0.35. Then, compute the product:

$$0.35 \times 5,600 = 1,960$$

Therefore, it would be expected that 1,960 of those commuters would speed on their way to work based on the data given. In this situation, the word "of" signals to use multiplication to find the answer. Another way percentages are used is in the following problem: Teachers work 8 months out of the year. What percent of the year do they work? To answer this problem, find what percent of 12 the number 8 is, because there are 12 months in a year. Therefore, divide 8 by 12, and convert that number to a percentage:

$$\frac{8}{12} = \frac{2}{3} = 0.66\bar{6}$$

The percentage rounded to the nearest tenth place tells us that teachers work 66.7% of the year. Percentage problems can also find missing quantities like in the following question: 60% of what number is 75? To find the missing quantity, turn the question into an equation. Let x be equal to the missing quantity. Therefore, $0.60x = 75$. Divide each side by 0.60 to isolate the variable. This yields $x = 125$. Therefore, 60% of 125 is equal to 75.

Sales tax is an important application relating to percentages because tax rates are usually given as percentages. For example, a city might have an 8% sales tax rate. Therefore, when an item is purchased with that tax rate, the real cost to the customer is 1.08 times the price in the store. For example, a $25 pair of jeans costs the customer:

$$\$25 \times 1.08 = \$27$$

If the sales tax rates is unknown, it can be determined after an item is purchased. If a customer visits a store and purchases an item for $21.44, but the price in the store was $19, they can find the tax rate by first subtracting:

$$\$21.44 - \$19$$

to obtain $2.44, the sales tax amount. The sales tax is a percentage of the in-store price. Therefore, the tax rate is:

$$\frac{2.44}{19} = 0.128$$

which has been rounded to the nearest thousandths place. In this scenario, the actual sales tax rate given as a percentage is 12.8%.

12-Hour Clock versus Military Time

There are two different methods of telling time. The first is the 24-hour clock, or what is sometimes called **military time**. This method is shown in the format hours:minutes. The current time is the number of hours and minutes past midnight. The other main way of telling time is the use of the 12-hour clock or the AM/PM system. This takes the 24 hours in a day and divides it into the nighttime hours, which run from midnight to noon, and the daytime hours, which run from noon to midnight. The hours from midnight to noon are the AM hours, and the hours from noon to midnight are the PM hours. Rather than counting up to 24, this method counts from 1 to 12 twice in one day.

To convert between the two methods, the other important piece of information to know is that the first hour of the day in the 24-hour clock is midnight, which would read 0:00. For the AM hours starting at 1:00 AM, the two methods will yield the same time. 2:30 AM on the 12-hour clock will be the same as 2:30 in military time. However, between midnight and 1:00 AM on the 12-hour clock, 12 hours must be subtracted to convert between the two methods. For example, if it is 12:35 AM in the 12-hour clock system, then subtract 12 hours to get 00:35 hours in military time. Conversely, if it is after noon, add 12 hours to the 12-hour clock time to get the military time. For example, if it is 3:15 PM by the 12-hour clock, add 12 hours to get 15:15 in military time.

Algebra

An **equation in one variable** is a mathematical statement where two algebraic expressions in one variable, usually x, are set equal. To solve the equation, the variable must be isolated on one side of the equals sign. The addition and multiplication principles of equality are used to isolate the variable. The **addition principle of equality** states that the same number can be added to or subtracted from both sides of an equation. Because the same value is being used on both sides of the equals sign, equality is maintained.

For example, the equation $2x - 3 = 5x$ is equivalent to both:

$$2x - 3 + 3 = 5x + 3$$

and

$$2x - 3 - 5 = 5x - 5$$

This principle can be used to solve the following equation: $x + 5 = 4$. The variable x must be isolated, so to move the 5 from the left side, subtract 5 from both sides of the equals sign. Therefore:

$$x + 5 - 5 = 4 - 5$$

So, the solution is $x = -1$. This process illustrates the idea of an **additive inverse** because subtracting 5 is the same as adding -5. Basically, add the opposite of the number that must be removed to both sides of the equals sign.

The **multiplication principle of equality** states that equality is maintained when a number is either multiplied by both expressions on each side of the equals sign, or when both expressions are divided by the same number. For example, $4x = 5$ is equivalent to both $16x = 20$ and $x = \frac{5}{4}$. Multiplying both sides by 4 and dividing both sides by 4 maintains equality. Solving the equation $6x - 18 = 5$ requires the use of both principles. First, the addition principle is applied by adding 18 to both sides of the equals sign, which results in $6x = 23$. Then the multiplication principle is used to divide both sides by 6, giving the solution $x = \frac{23}{6}$. Using the multiplication principle in the solving process is the same as involving a multiplicative inverse. A **multiplicative inverse** is a value that, when multiplied by a given number, results in 1. Dividing by 6 is the same as multiplying by $\frac{1}{6}$, which is both the reciprocal and multiplicative inverse of 6.

When solving a linear equation in one variable, checking the answer shows if the solution process was performed correctly. Plug the solution into the variable in the original equation. If the result is a false statement, something was done incorrectly during the solution procedure. Checking the example above gives the following:

$$6 \times \frac{23}{6} - 18 = 23 - 18 = 5$$

Therefore, the solution is correct.

Some equations in one variable involve fractions or the use of the distributive property. In either case, the goal is to obtain only one variable term and then use the addition and multiplication principles to isolate that variable. Consider the equation:

$$\frac{2}{3}x = 6$$

To solve for x, multiply each side of the equation by the reciprocal of $\frac{2}{3}$, which is $\frac{3}{2}$. This step results in $\frac{3}{2} \times \frac{2}{3}x = \frac{3}{2} \times 6$, which simplifies into the solution $x = 9$. Now consider the equation:

$$3(x + 2) - 5x = 4x + 1$$

The distributive property can be used to clear the parentheses. Therefore, each term inside the parentheses is multiplied by 3. This step results in:

$$3x + 6 - 5x = 4x + 1$$

Next, like terms are collected on the left-hand side. **Like terms** are terms with the same variable or variables raised to the same exponent(s). Only like terms can be combined through addition or subtraction. After collecting like terms, the equation is:

$$-2x + 6 = 4x + 1$$

Finally, the addition and multiplication principles are applied. $2x$ is added to both sides to obtain:

$$6 = 6x + 1$$

Then, 1 is subtracted from both sides to obtain $5 = 6x$. Finally, both sides are divided by 6 to obtain the solution $\frac{5}{6} = x$.

Two other types of solutions can be obtained when solving an equation in one variable. The final result could be that there is either no solution or that the solution set contains all real numbers. Consider the equation:

$$4x = 6x + 5 - 2x$$

First, the like terms can be combined on the right to obtain:

$$4x = 4x + 5$$

Next, $4x$ is subtracted from both sides. This step results in the false statement $0 = 5$. There is no value that can be plugged into x that will ever make this equation true. Therefore, there is no solution. The solution procedure contained correct steps, but the result of a false statement means that no value satisfies the equation. The symbolic way to denote that no solution exists is ∅. Next, consider the equation:

$$5x + 4 + 2x = 9 + 7x - 5$$

Combining the like terms on both sides results in:

$$7x + 4 = 7x + 4$$

The left-hand side is exactly the same as the right-hand side. Using the addition principle to move terms, the result is $0 = 0$, which is always true. Therefore, the original equation is true for any number, and the solution set is all real numbers. The symbolic way to denote such a solution set is $\mathbb{R}$, or in interval notation, $(-\infty, \infty)$.

One-step problems take only one mathematical step to solve. For example, solving the equation $5x = 45$ is a one-step problem because the one step of dividing both sides of the equation by 5 is the only step necessary to obtain the solution $x = 9$. The multiplication principle of equality is the one step used to isolate the variable. The equation is of the form $ax = b$, where a and b are rational numbers. Similarly, the addition principle of equality could be the one step needed to solve a problem. In this case, the equation would be of the form $x + a = b$ or $x - a = b$, for real numbers a and b.

A multi-step problem requires more than one step to find the solution, or it could consist of solving more than one equation. An equation that involves both the addition principle and the multiplication principle is a two-step problem, and an example of such an equation is:

$$2x - 4 = 5$$

Solving involves adding 4 to both sides and then dividing both sides by 2. An example of a two-step problem involving two separate equations is $y = 3x, 2x + y = 4$. The two equations form a system of two equations that must be solved together in two variables. The system can be solved by the substitution method. Since y is already solved for in terms of x, plug $3x$ in for y into the equation $2x + y = 4$, resulting in:

$$2x + 3x = 4$$

Therefore, $5x = 4$ and $x = \frac{4}{5}$. Because there are two variables, the solution consists of both a value for x and for y. To solve for y, $x = \frac{4}{5}$ is substituted into either original equation. The easiest choice is $y = 3x$. Therefore:

$$y = 3 \times \frac{4}{5} = \frac{12}{5}$$

The solution can be written as the ordered pair $\left(\frac{4}{5}, \frac{12}{5}\right)$.

Real-world problems can be translated into both one-step and multi-step problems. In either case, the word problem must be translated from the verbal form into mathematical expressions and equations that can be solved using algebra. An example of a one-step real-world problem is the following: A cat weighs half as much as a dog living in the same house. If the dog weighs 14.5 pounds, how much does the cat weigh? To solve this problem, an equation can be used. In any word problem, the first step must be defining variables that represent the unknown quantities. For this problem, let x be equal to the unknown weight of the cat. Because two times the weight of the cat equals 14.5 pounds, the equation to be solved is: $2x = 14.5$. Use the multiplication principle to divide both sides by 2. Therefore, $x = 7.25$. The cat weighs 7.25 pounds.

Most of the time, real-world problems are more difficult than this one and consist of multi-step problems. The following is an example of a multi-step problem: The sum of two consecutive page numbers is equal to 437. What are those page numbers? First, define the unknown quantities. If x is equal to the first page number, then $x + 1$ is equal to the next page number because they are consecutive integers. Their sum is equal to 437, and this statement translates to the equation:

$$x + x + 1 = 437$$

To solve, first collect like terms to obtain:

$$2x + 1 = 437$$

Then, subtract 1 from both sides and then divide by 2. The solution to the equation is $x = 218$. Therefore, the two consecutive page numbers that satisfy the problem are 218 and 219. It is always important to make sure that answers to real-world problems make sense. For instance, if the solution to this same problem resulted in decimals, that should be a red flag indicating the need to check the work. Page numbers are whole numbers; therefore, if decimals are found to be answers, the solution process should be double-checked to see where mistakes were made.

When presented with a real-world problem that must be solved, the first step is always to determine what the unknown quantity is that must be solved for. Use a variable, such as x or t, to represent that unknown quantity. Sometimes there can be two or more unknown quantities. In this case, either choose an additional variable, or if a relationship exists between the unknown quantities, express the other quantities in terms of the original variable. After choosing the variables, form algebraic expressions and/or equations that represent the verbal statement in the problem. The following table shows examples of vocabulary used to represent the different operations.

Addition	Sum, plus, total, increase, more than, combined, in all
Subtraction	Difference, less than, subtract, reduce, decrease, fewer, remain
Multiplication	Product, multiply, times, part of, twice, triple
Division	Quotient, divide, split, each, equal parts, per, average, shared

The combination of operations and variables form both mathematical expression and equations. The difference between expressions and equations are that there is no equals sign in an expression, and that expressions are *evaluated* to find an unknown quantity, while equations are *solved* to find an unknown quantity.

Measurement and Roman Numerals

When working with dimensions, sometimes the given units don't match the formula, and conversions must be made. The metric system has base units of meter for length, kilogram for mass, and liter for liquid volume. This system expands to three places above the base unit and three places below. These places correspond with prefixes with a base of 10. The following table shows the conversions:

kilo-	hecto-	deka-	base	deci-	centi-	milli-
1,000 times the base	100 times the base	10 times the base		1/10 times the base	1/100 times the base	1/1000 times the base

To convert between units within the metric system, values with a base ten can be multiplied. The decimal can also be moved in the direction of the new unit by the same number of zeros on the number. For example, 3 meters is equivalent to 0.003 kilometers. The decimal moved three places (the same number of zeros for kilo-) to the left (the same direction from base to kilo-). Three meters is also equivalent to 3,000 millimeters. The decimal is moved three places to the right because the prefix milli- is three places to the right of the base unit.

The English Standard system used in the United States has a base unit of foot for length, pound for weight, and gallon for liquid volume. Conversions within the English Standard system are not as easy as those within the metric system because the former does not use a base ten model. The following table shows the conversions within this system:

Length	Weight	Capacity
1 foot (ft) = 12 inches (in) 1 yard (yd) = 3 feet 1 mile (mi) = 5280 feet 1 mile = 1760 yards	1 pound (lb) = 16 ounces (oz) 1 ton = 2000 pounds	1 tablespoon (tbsp) = 3 teaspoons (tsp) 1 cup (c) = 16 tablespoons 1 cup = 8 fluid ounces (oz) 1 pint (pt) = 2 cups 1 quart (qt) = 2 pints 1 gallon (gal) = 4 quarts

When converting within the English Standard system, most calculations include a conversion to the base unit and then another to the desired unit. For example, take the following problem:

$$3 \text{ qt} = \underline{\quad} \text{ c}$$

There is no straight conversion from quarts to cups, so the first conversion is from quarts to pints. There are 2 pints in 1 quart, so there are 6 pints in 3 quarts. This conversion can be solved as a proportion:

$$\frac{3 \text{ qt}}{x} = \frac{1 \text{ qt}}{2 \text{ pt}}$$

It can also be observed as a ratio 2:1, expanded to 6:3. Then the 6 pints must be converted to cups. The ratio of pints to cups is 1:2, so the expanded ratio is 6:12. For 6 pints, the measurement is 12 cups. This problem can also be set up as one set of fractions to cancel out units. It begins with the given information and cancels out matching units on top and bottom to yield the answer. Consider the following expression:

$$\frac{3 \text{ qt}}{1} \times \frac{2 \text{ pt}}{1 \text{ qt}} \times \frac{2 \text{ c}}{1 \text{ pt}}$$

It's set up so that units on the top and bottom cancel each other out:

$$\frac{3 \ \cancel{\text{qt}}}{1} \times \frac{2 \ \cancel{\text{pt}}}{1 \ \cancel{\text{qt}}} \times \frac{2 \text{ c}}{1 \ \cancel{\text{pt}}}$$

The numbers can be calculated as $3 \times 2 \times 2$ on the top and 1 on the bottom. It still yields an answer of 12 cups.

This process of setting up fractions and canceling out matching units can be used to convert between standard and metric systems. A few common equivalent conversions are:

$$2.54 \text{ cm} = 1 \text{ in}$$

$$3.28 \text{ ft} = 1 \text{ m}$$

and

$$2.205 \text{ lb} = 1 \text{ kg}$$

Writing these as fractions allows them to be used in conversions. For the problem 5 meters = ___ ft, use the feet-to-meter conversion and start with the expression $\frac{5 \text{ m}}{1} \times \frac{3.28 \text{ ft}}{1 \text{ m}}$. The "meters" will cancel each other out, leaving "feet" as the final unit. Calculating the numbers yields 16.4 feet. This problem only required two fractions. Others may require longer expressions, but the underlying rule stays the same. When a unit in the numerator of a fraction matches a unit in the denominator, then they cancel each other out. Using this logic and the conversions given above, many units can be converted between and within the different systems.

The conversion between Fahrenheit and Celsius temperature is found in a formula:

$$°C = (°F - 32) \times \frac{5}{9}$$

For example, to convert 78°F to Celsius, the given temperature would be entered into the formula:

$$°C = (78 - 32) \times \frac{5}{9}$$

Solving the equation, the temperature comes out to be 25.56°C. To convert in the other direction, the formula becomes:

$$°F = °C * \frac{9}{5} + 32$$

Remember the order of operations when calculating these conversions.

Roman numerals are sometimes used in place of Arabic numbers. The Roman numeral system uses different letter combinations to represent numbers. Seven letters are utilized in this system. The chart below shows the more common numerals and what number they indicate:

Roman Numeral	Number Equivalent	Roman Numeral	Number Equivalent
I	1	XX	20
II	2	XXX	30
III	3	XL	40
IV	4	L	50
V	5	LX	60
VI	6	LXX	70
VII	7	LXXX	80
VIII	8	XC	90
IX	9	C	100
X	10	D	500
XI	11	M	1000

There are rules for the different combinations. When a symbol comes after a symbol for a larger number, it is added to the larger symbol. If a symbol appears before a symbol or a larger number, then it should be subtracted. For example, XXXIV represents 34 because:

$$10 + 10 + 10 + 5 - 1 = 34$$

For larger Roman numerals, a dash is added to the top of the symbol that indicates times 1,000. For example, $\overline{X}$ equals 10,000 because:

$$10 \times 1,000 = 10,000$$

Helpful Information to Memorize

In addition to the list of Roman Numerals, measurement conversions, and formulas presented in the previous sections, prepared test takers commit to memory several key mathematical formulas. Questions in the Math section of the HESI A2 may require knowledge of certain formulas in order to correctly obtain the answer. Other questions can be answered much more quickly if conversions that *can* be calculated out are instead readily available in stored memory. Time saved by not having to perform calculations to obtain an answer can be allocated to more difficult questions that may otherwise not receive ample time to solve. For example, it is common to encounter a fraction, such as 2/5, that must be converted to a decimal or percentage. Instead of calculating the answer by hand or via calculator, test takers who have committed to memory these conversions for basic values such as this one, can automatically select the correct answer of 0.40 or 40% and then quickly move on the next question.

In addition to temperature conversions, Roman Numerals, and the common measurements previously listed, the following simple equivalencies should be memorized for a better experience on test day:

Fraction	Decimal	Percent
1/2	0.50	50%
1/3	0.333	33.3%
1/4	0.25	25%
1/5	0.20	20%
1/6	0.166	16.6%
1/8	0.125	12.5%

Approximate Measurement Conversions	
1 inch	2.54 cm
1 cm	0.39 inches
1 mile	1.61 kms
1 km	0.62 miles

HESI Math Practice Questions

1. $10.62 + 4.39 =$
   a. 14.91
   b. 14.01
   c. 15.01
   d. 5.01

2. $6.23 \times 4.5 =$
   a. 28.035
   b. 5.607
   c. 280.35
   d. 28.025

3. $1,289 - 356 =$
   a. 833
   b. 933
   c. 924
   d. 856

4. $273 \div 7 =$
   a. 38
   b. 36
   c. 39
   d. 49

5. Which of the following expressions best exemplifies the distributive property?
   a. $(6 + 8) + 5 = 6 + (8 + 5)$
   b. $4 \times 6 \times 3 = 3 \times 6 \times 4$
   c. $9 \times 1 = 9$
   d. $4 \times (8 + 3) = 4 \times 8 + 4 \times 3$

6. $8 \times (6 + 2) - 4 \div 2 =$
   a. 30
   b. 16
   c. 64
   d. 62

7. $-6 \times (-9) \div 3 =$
   a. 21
   b. 18
   c. -21
   d. -18

8. What is $\frac{12}{60}$ converted to a percentage?
   a. 0.20
   b. 20%
   c. 25%
   d. 12%

9. Which of the following is the correct decimal form of the fraction $\frac{14}{33}$ rounded to the nearest hundredth place?

    a. 0.420

    b. 0.42

    c. 0.424

    d. 0.140

10. What is 1.56 converted to a simplified fraction?

    a. $1\frac{56}{100}$

    b. $1\frac{28}{50}$

    c. $1\frac{14}{25}$

    d. $\frac{28}{50}$

11. Which of the following represents the correct sum of $\frac{14}{15}$ and $\frac{2}{5}$, in lowest possible terms?

    a. $\frac{20}{15}$

    b. $\frac{4}{3}$

    c. $\frac{16}{20}$

    d. $\frac{4}{5}$

12. What is the product of $\frac{5}{14}$ and $\frac{7}{20}$?

    a. $\frac{1}{8}$

    b. $\frac{35}{280}$

    c. $\frac{12}{34}$

    d. $\frac{1}{2}$

13. What is the result of dividing 24 by $\frac{8}{5}$?

    a. $\frac{5}{3}$

    b. $\frac{3}{5}$

    c. $\frac{120}{8}$

    d. 15

14. Subtract $\frac{5}{14}$ from $\frac{5}{24}$. Which of the following is the correct result?
   a. $\frac{25}{168}$
   b. 0
   c. $-\frac{25}{168}$
   d. $\frac{1}{10}$

15. A jar is filled with green, yellow, and orange marbles. If $\frac{1}{4}$ of the marbles are green and $\frac{2}{7}$ are yellow, what fraction of the marbles are orange?
   a. $\frac{15}{28}$
   b. $\frac{13}{28}$
   c. $\frac{2}{3}$
   d. $\frac{3}{7}$

16. What is the solution to the equation $3(x + 2) = 14x - 5$?
   a. $x = 1$
   b. No solution
   c. $x = 0$
   d. All real numbers

17. What is the solution to the equation $10 - 5x + 2 = 7x + 12 - 12x$?
   a. $x = 12$
   b. No solution
   c. $x = 0$
   d. All real numbers

18. Which of the following is the result when solving the equation $4(x + 5) + 6 = 2(2x + 3)$?
   a. Any real number is a solution.
   b. There is no solution.
   c. $x = 6$ is the solution.
   d. $x = 26$ is the solution.

19. How many cases of cola can Lexi purchase if each case is $3.50 and she has $40?
   a. 10
   b. 12
   c. 11.4
   d. 11

20. Two consecutive integers exist such that the sum of three times the first and two less than the second is equal to 411. What are those integers?
   a. 103 and 104
   b. 104 and 105
   c. 102 and 103
   d. 100 and 101

21. In a neighborhood, 15 out of 80 of the households have children under the age of 18. What percentage of the households have children under 18?

    a. 0.1875%

    b. 18.75%

    c. 1.875%

    d. 15%

22. Gina took an algebra test last Friday. There were 35 questions, and she answered 60% of them correctly. How many correct answers did she have?

    a. 35

    b. 20

    c. 21

    d. 25

23. Paul took a written driving test, and he got 12 of the questions correct. If he answered 75% of the total questions correctly, how many problems were on the test?

    a. 25

    b. 16

    c. 20

    d. 18

24. If a car is purchased for $15,395 with a 7.25% sales tax, how much is the total price?

    a. $15,395.07

    b. $16,511.14

    c. $16,411.13

    d. $15,402

25. Bindee is having a barbeque on Sunday and needs 12 packets of ketchup for every 5 guests. If 60 guests are coming, how many packets of ketchup should she buy?

    a. 100

    b. 12

    c. 144

    d. 60

26. A grocery store sold 48 bags of apples in one day. If 9 of the bags contained Granny Smith apples and the rest contained Red Delicious apples, what is the ratio of bags of Granny Smith to bags of Red Delicious that were sold?

    a. 48:9

    b. 39:9

    c. 9:48

    d. 9:39

27. If Oscar's bank account totaled $4,000 in March and $4,900 in June, what was the rate of change in his bank account total over those three months?

    a. $900 a month

    b. $300 a month

    c. $4,900 a month

    d. $100 a month

28. How many kiloliters are in 6 liters?
    a. 6,000
    b. 600
    c. 0.006
    d. 0.0006

29. How many centimeters are in 3 feet? (Note: 2.54 cm = 1 in)
    a. 0.635
    b. 91.44
    c. 14.17
    d. 7.62

30. If Sandy can bike 8 miles in 25 minutes, how many miles can she bike in 55 minutes?
    a. 17.6 miles
    b. 16 miles
    c. 16.9 miles
    d. 17.3 miles

31. What is 17:53 in military time converted to standard time?
    a. 5:53 PM
    b. 5:53 AM
    c. 7:53 AM
    d. 7:53 PM

32. What is 3:35 PM converted to military time?
    a. 13:35
    b. 15:35
    c. 9:35
    d. 5:35

33. A nurse arrives at work at 18:00 for a 10-hour shift. What time does her shift end?
    a. 6 PM
    b. 6 AM
    c. 2 AM
    d. 4 AM

34. What is the solution to the following system of equations?
$$14 = 3x + 2y$$
$$y = 2x$$
    a. (4, 2)
    b. (3, 4)
    c. (2, 4)
    d. (2, 6)

35. What algebraic expression represents the following phrase?
    The sum of nine and the product of 3 and a number x.
    a. $9 \times 3x$
    b. $(3 + 9)x$
    c. $(3 \times 9) + x$
    d. $9 + 3x$

36. Emma bought four notebooks at $2.50 each and 3 boxes of pencils at $1.35 each. If she gave the cashier a $20 bill, how much change should she receive?
   a. $7.30
   b. $5.95
   c. $3.45
   d. $14.05

37. A patient has been instructed to drink a gallon of water each day. How many cups does the patient need to drink?
   a. 16 cups
   b. 8 cups
   c. 24 cups
   d. 12 cups

38. The temperature at Sam's house was 95°F. What was the temperature in Celsius?
   a. 63°C
   b. 113°C
   c. 20°C
   d. 35°C

39. When the temperature reaches 100°F, the children at the local pool must get out. The current temperature is 30°C. How many °F can the temperature climb before the children must get out?
   a. 37
   b. 86
   c. 14
   d. 8

40. The number 1236 is equivalent to which Roman numeral?
   a. MCXXXVI
   b. MCCXXVI
   c. MCCXXXVI
   d. MCCXXXIV

41. The Roman numeral CCLIX is equivalent to which Arabic number?
   a. 259
   b. 2059
   c. 2509
   d. 2511

42. $6 + 10.24 + 3.021 =$
   a. 19.45
   b. 19.261
   c. 20.261
   d. 19.36

43. Andrea has 6 black shirts, 8 white shirts, 5 red shirts, 4 blue shirts, and 7 gray shirts. If 40% of her shirts have long sleeves, how many have short sleeves?

    a. 12

    b. 18

    c. 19

    d. 16

44. There are 99 boys per every 3 grade levels at a local high school. How many boys are there in 7 grade levels?

    a. 297

    b. 252

    c. 226

    d. 231

45. A jewelry store sells bracelets, necklaces, rings, and earrings. Each type of jewelry has several models. The number of models and sales amount per day are listed in the following table:

Type of Jewelry	Models	Amount Sold of Each Model per Day
Bracelets	3	6
Necklaces	5	5
Rings	6	4
Earrings	8	5

How many pieces of jewelry are sold in a day?

    a. 20

    b. 97

    c. 22

    d. 107

46. Using the table from the previous question, what is the ratio of total necklaces sold to total earrings sold?

    a. 5:5

    b. 24:40

    c. 25:40

    d. 5:8

47. Jennifer makes $14.65 an hour and 20% of each sale she makes as her commission. If she works for 8 hours and makes a total of $273.20 in a day, what were her total sales for the day?

    a. $54.64

    b. $780

    c. $156

    d. $586

48. $\frac{1}{2}\left(\frac{1}{4} + \frac{5}{8}\right) =$

    a. $\frac{7}{16}$

    b. $\frac{7}{8}$

    c. $\frac{9}{16}$

    d. $\frac{11}{8}$

49. What is the value of y in the following equation, if $x = -4$?

$$y = 3x - 6x + 8$$

    a. 20
    b. -28
    c. 44
    d. 32

50. 12 is what percentage of 80?
    a. 12%
    b. 8%
    c. 15%
    d. 6%

51. A car manufacturer usually makes 15,412 SUVs, 25,815 station wagons, 50,412 sedans, 8,123 trucks, and 18,312 hybrids a month. About how many cars are manufactured each month?
    a. 120,000
    b. 200,000
    c. 300,000
    d. 12,000

52. Each year, a family goes to the grocery store every week and spends $105. About how much does the family spend annually on groceries?
    a. $10,000
    b. $50,000
    c. $500
    d. $5,000

53. Triple the difference of five and a number is equal to the sum of that number and 5. What is the number?
    a. 5
    b. 2
    c. 5.5
    d. 2.5

54. In order to estimate deer population in a forest, biologists obtained a sample of deer in that forest and tagged each one of them. The sample had 300 deer in total. They returned a week later and harmlessly captured 400 deer, and found that 5 were tagged. Using this information, which of the following is the best estimate of the total number of deer in the forest?

    a. 24,000 deer

    b. 30,000 deer

    c. 40,000 deer

    d. 100,000 deer

55. The number of members of the House of Representatives varies directly with the total population in a state. If the state of New York has 19,800,000 residents and has 27 total representatives, how many should Ohio have with a population of 11,800,000?

    a. 10

    b. 16

    c. 11

    d. 5

56. A thermometer currently reads 37°C. What is this temperature in Fahrenheit?

    a. 84.6°F

    b. 34.6°F

    c. 98.6°F

    d. 52.6°F

57. At a certain hospital, the ratio of nurses to patients is 1:3. If the hospital has 99 patients, how many nurses are working?

    a. 33

    b. 297

    c. 25

    d. 17

58. A saline solution has 18 grams of salt for every 2 liters of water. How many grams of salt are needed for 9 liters of water?

    a. 1 g

    b. 81 g

    c. 162 g

    d. 18 g

59. A baby was born weighing 7 pounds and 12 ounces. What is their weight in kilograms to the nearest tenth? (There are 28.35 grams in one ounce.)

    a. 3.8 kg

    b. 2.8 kg

    c. 3.5 kg

    d. 3.6 kg

60. In a critical care unit, there are 45 beds and 27 patients. What is the ratio of patients to beds expressed in simplest terms?

    a. 27:45
    b. 9:15
    c. 5:3
    d. 3:5

Answer Explanations

1. C: The first step is to line the decimal points up, and then add the numbers vertically.

$$10^1.6^12$$
$$+ \quad 4.39$$
$$\overline{15.01}$$

2. A: To complete this problem, first remove the decimals. Next, complete the multiplication to find the product, 28,035. Because there are three decimal places in the original problem, the decimal needs to be placed three places to the left. This gives a solution of 28.035.

3. B: The numbers must be lined up so that the place value lines up vertically. Then, subtract accordingly.

$$^0\!\not{1}^1289$$
$$- \quad 356$$
$$\overline{933}$$

4. C: The division problem is completed as follows.

$$\begin{array}{r} 39 \\ 7\overline{)273} \\ 21\downarrow \\ \overline{63} \\ 63 \\ \overline{0} \end{array}$$

5. D: The distributive property is used when a number is being multiplied by a term or terms inside of parentheses. The number outside the parentheses is multiplied, or distributed, to each term, and the results are added or subtracted as called for.

6. D: To solve this expression, the order of operations must be used. The first step is to evaluate what is inside the parentheses:

$$8 \times (8) - 4 \div 2$$

Next, the multiplication and division should be completed: $64 - 2$. The last step is to subtract,

$$64 - 2 = 62$$

7. B: The rule of negative numbers states that if two negative numbers are multiplied together, the resulting product is positive. Therefore:

$$-6 \times (-9) = 54$$

Then, 54 can be divided by 3 to find the answer of 18.

8. B: The fraction $\frac{12}{60}$ can be reduced to $\frac{1}{5}$, in lowest terms. First, it must be converted to a decimal. Dividing 1 by 5 results in 0.2. Then, to convert to a percentage, move the decimal point two units to the right and add the percentage symbol. The result is 20%.

9. B: If a calculator is used, divide 33 into 14 and keep two decimal places. If a calculator is not used, multiply both the numerator and denominator by 3. This results in the fraction $\frac{42}{99}$, and hence a decimal of 0.42.

10. C: The decimal portion of 1.56 must be placed over 100 which yields $1\frac{56}{100}$. However, this can be further simplified. The fraction portion can be reduced by a factor of 4. The result is $1\frac{14}{25}$.

11. B: Common denominators must be used. The LCD is 15, and $\frac{2}{5} = \frac{6}{15}$. Therefore, $\frac{14}{15} + \frac{6}{15} = \frac{20}{15}$, and in lowest terms, the answer is $\frac{4}{3}$. A common factor of 5 was divided out of both the numerator and denominator.

12. A: A product is found by multiplication. Multiplying two fractions together is easier when common factors are cancelled first to avoid working with larger numbers.

$$\frac{5}{14} \times \frac{7}{20} = \frac{5}{2 \cdot 7} \times \frac{7}{5 \cdot 4}$$

$$\frac{1}{2} \times \frac{1}{4} = \frac{1}{8}$$

13. D: Division is completed by multiplying by the reciprocal. Therefore:

$$24 \div \frac{8}{5} = \frac{24}{1} \times \frac{5}{8}$$

$$\frac{3 \cdot 8}{1} \times \frac{5}{8} = \frac{15}{1} = 15$$

14. C: Common denominators must be used. The LCD is 168, so each fraction must be converted to have 168 as the denominator.

$$\frac{5}{24} - \frac{5}{14} = \frac{5}{24} \times \frac{7}{7} - \frac{5}{14} \times \frac{12}{12}$$

$$\frac{35}{168} - \frac{60}{168} = -\frac{25}{168}$$

15. B: The total fraction of green and yellow marbles is:

$$\frac{1}{4} + \frac{2}{7} = \frac{7}{28} + \frac{8}{28} = \frac{15}{28}$$

The fraction of orange marbles is:

$$1 - \frac{15}{28} = \frac{28}{28} - \frac{15}{28} = \frac{13}{28}$$

16. A: First, the distributive property must be used on the left side. This results in:

$$3x + 6 = 14x - 5$$

The addition principle is then used to add 5 to both sides, and then to subtract $3x$ from both sides, resulting in $11 = 11x$. Finally, the multiplication principle is used to divide each side by 11. Therefore, $x = 1$ is the solution.

17. D: First, like terms are collected to obtain:

$$12 - 5x = -5x + 12$$

Then, the addition principle is used to move the terms with the variable, so $5x$ is added to both sides and the mathematical statement $12 = 12$ is obtained. This is always true; therefore, all real numbers satisfy the original equation.

18. B: The distributive property is used on both sides to obtain:

$$4x + 20 + 6 = 4x + 6$$

Then, like terms are collected on the left, resulting in:

$$4x + 26 = 4x + 6$$

Next, the addition principle is used to subtract $4x$ from both sides, and this results in the false statement $26 = 6$. Therefore, there is no solution.

19. D: This is a one-step real-world application problem. The unknown quantity is the number of cases of cola to be purchased. Let x be equal to this amount. Because each case costs $3.50, the total number of cases multiplied by $3.50 must equal $40. This translates to the mathematical equation $3.5x = 40$. Divide both sides by 3.5 to obtain $x = 11.4286$, which has been rounded to four decimal places. Because cases are sold whole, and there is not enough money to purchase 12 cases, 11 cases is the correct answer.

20. A: First, the variables have to be defined. Let x be the first integer; therefore, $x + 1$ is the second integer. This is a two-step problem. The sum of three times the first and two less than the second is translated into the following expression:

$$3x + (x + 1 - 2)$$

This expression is set equal to 411 to obtain

$$3x + (x + 1 - 2) = 411$$

The left-hand side is simplified to obtain $4x - 1 = 411$. The addition and multiplication properties are used to solve for x. First, add 1 to both sides and then divide both sides by 4 to obtain $x = 103$. The next consecutive integer is 104.

21. B: First, the information is translated into the ratio $\frac{15}{80}$. To find the percentage, translate this fraction into a decimal by dividing 15 by 80. The corresponding decimal is 0.1875. Move the decimal point two units to the right to obtain the percentage 18.75%.

22. C: Gina answered 60% of 35 questions correctly; 60% can be expressed as the decimal 0.60. Therefore, she answered $0.60 \times 35 = 21$ questions correctly.

23. B: The unknown quantity is the number of total questions on the test. Let x be equal to this unknown quantity. Therefore, $0.75x = 12$. Divide both sides by 0.75 to obtain $x = 16$.

24. B: If sales tax is 7.25%, the price of the car must be multiplied by 1.0725 to account for the additional sales tax. This is the same as multiplying the initial price by 0.0725 (the tax) and adding that to the initial cost. Therefore:

$$15,395 \times 1.0725 = 16,511.1375$$

This amount is rounded to the nearest cent, which is $16,511.14.

25. C: This problem involves ratios and percentages. If 12 packets are needed for every 5 people, this statement is equivalent to the ratio $\frac{12}{5}$. The unknown amount x is the number of ketchup packets needed for 60 people. The proportion $\frac{12}{5} = \frac{x}{60}$ must be solved. Cross-multiply to obtain:

$$12 \times 60 = 5x$$

Therefore, $720 = 5x$. Divide each side by 5 to obtain $x = 144$.

26. D: There were 48 total bags of apples sold. If 9 bags were Granny Smith and the rest were Red Delicious, then $48 - 9 = 39$ bags were Red Delicious. Therefore, the ratio of Granny Smith to Red Delicious is 9:39.

27. B: The average rate of change is found by calculating the difference in dollars over the elapsed time. Therefore, the rate of change is equal to ($4,900 - $4,000) ÷ 3 months, which is equal to $900 ÷ 3 or $300 per month.

28. C: There are 0.006 kiloliters in 6 liters because 1 liter is 0.001 kiloliters. The conversion comes from the metric prefix -kilo which has a value of 1000. Thus, 1 kiloliter is 1000 liters, and 1 liter is 0.001 kiloliters.

29. B: The conversion between feet and centimeters requires a middle term. As there are 2.54 centimeters in 1 inch, the conversion between inches and feet must be found. As there are 12 inches in a foot, the fractions can be set up as follows:

$$3 \text{ ft} \times \frac{12 \text{ in}}{1 \text{ ft}} \times \frac{2.54 \text{ cm}}{1 \text{ in}}$$

The feet and inches cancel out to leave only centimeters for the answer. The numbers are calculated across the top and bottom to yield:

$$\frac{3 \times 12 \times 2.54}{1 \times 1} = 91.44$$

The number and units used together form the answer of 91.44 cm.

30. A: To solve the problem, a proportion is created using ratios to compare distance and time. The proportion $\frac{8}{25} = \frac{x}{55}$ is used to find the missing distance. The ratios are cross multiplied to find the answer. $25x = 55 \times 8$, which becomes $25x = 440$. Solve for x to find $x = 17.6$.

31. A: To convert military time to the 12-hour clock system, 12 hours must be subtracted from 17:53 to find 5:53. The time is PM because the hours from 12 to 24 in the military time system are equivalent to the PM, or daytime hours, in the 12-hour clock system.

32. B: To convert standard time to military time, consider whether the standard time is PM or AM. If the time is PM, then 12 hours must be added.

33. D: 18:00 military time can be converted to standard time by subtracting 12 to give 6 PM. Starting at 6 PM, a 10-hour shift would end at 4 AM.

34. C: To solve a system of equations, substitution is one method that can be used. Because one equation is already solved for a variable, $y = 2x$, can be substituted into:

$$14 = 3x + 2y$$

This results in the following equation:

$$14 = 3x + 2(2x) \rightarrow 14 = 3x + 4x$$

$$14 = 7x \rightarrow x = 2$$

Plug the value of x into $y = 2x$ to get:

$$y = 2(2) \rightarrow y = 4$$

35. D: The phrase can be broken down into parts to find the expression. The sum of indicates that the 9 and the product will be added together. The product of 3 and a number x can be translated into 3 times x. The resulting expression is $9 + 3x$.

36. B: The total amount spent must be calculated first. The total for the notebooks is $4 \times \$2.50 = \$10.00$, and the total for the boxes of pencils is:

$$3 \times \$1.35 = \$4.05$$

The sum of the two amounts is:

$$\$10.00 + \$4.05 = \$14.05$$

To find the amount of change received, subtract the sum from the amount paid:

$$\$20 - \$14.05 = \$5.95$$

37. A: A series of proportions can be set up to convert from gallons to cups.

$$\frac{4 \; quarts}{1 \; gallon} \times \frac{2 \; pints}{1 \; quart} \times \frac{2 \; cups}{1 \; pint} = \frac{16 \; cups}{1 \; gallon}$$

38. D: To convert Fahrenheit to Celsius, the following formula must be used:

$$°C = (°F - 32) \times \frac{5}{9}$$

Substituting 95°F into the formula yields:

$$(95 - 32) \times \frac{5}{9} = 35°C$$

39. C: The first step to solve the problem is to convert 30°C to Fahrenheit using the following formula:

$$°F = °C \times \frac{9}{5} + 32$$

The substitution yields:

$$30 \times \frac{9}{5} + 32 = 86°F$$

The difference between 100°F and 86°F is 14. This represents how much the temperature can rise before the children must get out of the pool.

40. C: To convert Arabic numbers to Roman numerals, the corresponding symbols must be used for each denomination. The symbol for 1,000 is M, C for 100, X for 10, and VI for 6. 1236 has 1, 1,000; 2, 100s; 3, 10's; and the 6 which combine to make MCCXXXVI.

41. A: To convert Roman numerals to Arabic numbers, the numbers must be substituted for the symbols. The C is for 100, the L is for 50, and the IX is for 9. Because there are 2 C's, the Arabic number is 259.

42. B: The first step is to line the decimal points up, and then add the numbers vertically. Because these numbers have different amounts of place value before and after the decimal, zeros will need to be added as placeholders.

$$
\begin{array}{r}
6.000 \\
10.240 \\
+\ 3.021 \\
\hline
19.261
\end{array}
$$

43. B: The total number of shirts Andrea has is:

$$6 + 8 + 5 + 4 + 7 = 30$$

If 40% of her shirts have long sleeves, then $100 - 40 = 60\%$ must have short sleeves. Because 60% is equivalent to .60, the total number of shirts, 30, can be multiplied by .60 to find the number of short sleeve shirts.

$$30 \times .60 = 18$$

44. D: This problem can be solved using proportions and ratios. If there are 99 boys for every 3 grade levels, this statement is equivalent to the ratio $\frac{99}{3}$. The unknown amount x is the number of boys in 7 grade levels. The proportion $\frac{99}{3} = \frac{x}{7}$ must be solved. Cross-multiply to obtain:

$$99 \times 7 = 3x$$

Therefore, $693 = 3x$. Divide each side by 3 to find the answer of $x = 231$.

45. D: The first step in this problem is to find how many of each item were sold in a day. To find this amount, the number of models (2nd column) must be multiplied by the number of each model sold (3rd column). Then, the products must be added together to get a final total:

$$(3 \times 6) + (5 \times 5) + (6 \times 4) + (8 \times 5) = 107$$

46. D: The ratio of total necklaces to total earrings can be found by setting the total number of necklaces, which is $5 \times 5 = 25$, before the ratio symbol. The total number of earrings, which is $8 \times 5 = 40$, is placed after the ratio symbol to create the ratio 25:40. This can be simplified to 5:8 by dividing both sides by 5.

47. B: An expression representing this situation can be used to find Jennifer's total amount of sales for the day. Let t be the total amount of money she made for the day, h be the hours she worked, and s be her sales for the day. The expression is as follows, substituting her hourly rate and her commission of 20% (.20):

$$t = 14.65 \times h + 0.2 \times s$$

Input the known values of the total money made in the day and the hours she worked. Then, the equation can be solved for s to find the sales for the day:

$$273.20 = 14.65 \times 8 + .20s$$

$$273.20 = 117.20 + .20s$$

$$156 = .20s$$

$$s = 780$$

48. A: The first step to solve this problem is to use the distributive property to multiply $\frac{1}{2}$ by the two terms inside the parentheses, which yields $\frac{1}{8} + \frac{5}{16}$. Next, a common denominator of 16 must be used before the two terms can be added together:

$$\frac{2}{16} + \frac{5}{16} = \frac{7}{16}$$

49. A: To find the value of y, substitute the value of x into the given equation and solve for y. The rules for multiplication of negative numbers must be used.

$$y = 3x - 6x + 8$$

$$y = 3(-4) - 6(-4) + 8$$

$$y = -12 + 24 + 8$$

$$y = 20$$

50. C: An equation can be used to find the correct percentage. Use $80x = 12$ to find the solution of $x = 0.15$. This can be converted to a percentage by moving the decimal two places to the right and adding the percent sign.

51. A: Rounding can be used to find the best approximation. All of the values can be rounded to the nearest thousand. 15,412 SUVs can be rounded to 15,000. 25,815 station wagons can be rounded to

26,000. 50,412 sedans can be rounded to 50,000. 8,123 trucks can be rounded to 8,000. Finally, 18,312 hybrids can be rounded to 18,000. The sum of the rounded values is 117,000, which is closest to 120,000.

52. D: There are 52 weeks in a year, and if the family spends $105 each week, that amount is close to $100. A good approximation is $100 a week for 50 weeks, which is found through the product:

$$50 \times \$100 = \$5,000$$

53. D: Let x be the unknown number. The difference indicates subtraction, and sum represents addition. To triple the difference, it is multiplied by 3. The problem can be expressed as the following equation:

$$3(5 - x) = x + 5$$

Distributing the 3 results in:

$$15 - 3x = x + 5$$

Subtract 5 from both sides, add $3x$ to both sides, and then divide both sides by 4. This results in:

$$x = \frac{10}{4} = \frac{5}{2} = 2.5$$

54. A: A proportion should be used to solve this problem. The ratio of tagged to total deer in each instance is set equal, and the unknown quantity is a variable x. The proportion is:

$$\frac{300}{x} = \frac{5}{400}$$

Cross-multiplying gives $120,000 = 5x$, and dividing through by 5 results in 24,000.

55. B: The number of representatives varies directly with the population, so the equation necessary is $N = k \times P$, where N is number of representatives, k is the variation constant, and P is total population in millions. Plugging in the information for New York allows k to be solved for. This process gives $27 = k \times 19.8$, so $k = 1.36$. Therefore, the formula for number of representatives given total population in millions is $N = 1.36 \times P$. Plugging in $P = 11.8$ for Ohio results in $N = 16.05$, which rounds to 16 total representatives.

56. C: Recall the conversion from Celsius to Fahrenheit temperature:

$$°F = °C * \frac{9}{5} + 32$$

Plugging in 37°C yields:

$$°F = 37 * \frac{9}{5} + 32$$

$$= 66.6 + 32$$

$$= 98.6$$

57. A: Set up the proportion to solve for the unknown quantity, the number of nurses working at a hospital with 99 patients:

$$\frac{1 \; nurse}{3 \; patients} = \frac{x}{99 \; patients}$$

43

Cross multiplying results in $99 = 3x$. Divide both sides by 3 to obtain $x = 33$.

58. B: Reducing the ratio of 18 grams of salt to 2 liters of water by 2 yields 9 grams of salt per liter of water. For 9 liters of water, you would need $9 \times 9 \ grams \ of \ salt = 81 \ grams \ of \ salt.$

Another way to solve is to set up a proportion and cross multiply:

$$\frac{18 \ grams \ of \ salt}{2 \ liters \ of \ water} = \frac{x}{9 \ liters \ of \ water}$$

This results in:

$$2x = 18 \times 9$$

$$2x = 162$$

$$x = 81 \ grams \ of \ salt$$

59. C: First, convert the weight from pounds and ounces to only ounces:

$$7 \ lbs \ 12 \ oz = \frac{7 \ lbs}{1} \times \frac{16 \ oz}{1 \ lb} + 12 \ oz$$

$$= 112 \ oz + 12 \ oz$$

$$= 124 \ oz$$

Next, using the information given, convert the weight in ounces to grams:

$$124 \ oz = \frac{124 \ oz}{1} \times \frac{28.35 \ g}{1 \ oz} = 3515.4 \ g$$

Finally, convert the weight from grams to kilograms and round to the tenths place:

$$3515.4 \ g = \frac{3515.4 \ g}{1} \times \frac{1 \ kg}{1000 \ g} = 3.5154 \ kg \approx 3.5 \ kg$$

60. D: The ratio of patients to beds would be $27:45$. This ratio can be reduced by dividing both parts by 9, yielding $3:5$.

Reading Comprehension

Identifying the Topic, Main Idea, and Supporting Details

The **topic** of a text is the general subject matter. Text topics can usually be expressed in one word, or a few words at most. Additionally, readers should ask themselves what point the author is trying to make. This point is the **main idea** or **primary purpose** of the text, the principal thing the author wants readers to know concerning the topic. Once the author has established the main idea, he or she will support the main idea by supporting details. Supporting details are evidence that support the main idea and include personal testimonies, examples, or statistics.

One analogy for these components and their relationships is that a text is like a well-designed house. The topic is the roof, covering all rooms. The main idea is the frame. The supporting details are the various rooms. To identify the topic of a text, readers can ask themselves what or who the author is writing about in the paragraph. To locate the main idea, readers can ask themselves what one idea the author wants readers to know about the topic. To identify supporting details, readers can put the main idea into question form and ask, "what does the author use to prove or explain their main idea?"

Let's look at an example. An author is writing an essay about the Amazon rainforest and trying to convince the audience that more funding should go into protecting the area from deforestation. The author makes the argument stronger by including evidence of the benefits of the rainforest: it provides habitats to a variety of species, it provides much of the earth's oxygen which in turn cleans the atmosphere, and it is the home to medicinal plants that may be the answer to some of the world's deadliest diseases. Here is an outline of the essay looking at topic, main idea, and supporting details:

- Topic: Amazon rainforest
- Main Idea: The Amazon rainforest should receive more funding to protect it from deforestation.
- Supporting Details:
    1. It provides habitats to a variety of species.
    2. It provides much of the earth's oxygen, which, in turn, cleans the atmosphere.
    3. It is home to medicinal plants that may treat some of the world's deadliest diseases.

Notice that the topic of the essay is listed in a few key words: "Amazon rainforest." The main idea tells us what about the topic is important: that the topic should be funded in order to prevent deforestation. Finally, the supporting details are what author relies on to convince the audience to act or to believe in the truth of the main idea.

Finding the Meaning of Words in Context

Readers can often figure out what unfamiliar words mean without interrupting their reading to look them up in dictionaries by examining context. Context includes the other words or sentences in a passage. One common context clue is the root word and any affixes (prefixes/suffixes). Another common context clue is a synonym or definition included in the sentence. Sometimes both exist in the same sentence. Here's an example:

Scientists who study birds are *ornithologists*.

Many readers may not know the word *ornithologist*. However, the example contains a definition (scientists who study birds). The reader may also have the ability to analyze the suffix (*-logy*, meaning the study of) and root (*ornitho-*, meaning bird).

Another common context clue is a sentence that shows differences. Here's an example:

Birds *incubate* their eggs outside of their bodies, unlike mammals.

Some readers may be unfamiliar with the word *incubate*. However, since we know that "unlike mammals," birds incubate their eggs outside of their bodies, we can infer that *incubate* has something to do with keeping eggs warm outside the body until they are hatched.

In addition to analyzing the etymology of a word's root and affixes and extrapolating word meaning from sentences that contrast an unknown word with an antonym, readers can also determine word meanings from sentence context clues based on logic. Here's an example:

Birds are always looking out for *predators* that could attack their young.

The reader who is unfamiliar with the word *predator* could determine from the context of the sentence that predators usually prey upon baby birds and possibly other young animals. Readers might also use the context clue of etymology here, as *predator* and *prey* have the same root.

When readers encounter an unfamiliar word in text, they can use the surrounding context—the overall subject matter, specific chapter/section topic, and especially the immediate sentence context. Among others, one category of context clues is grammar. For example, the position of a word in a sentence and its relationship to the other words can help the reader establish whether the unfamiliar word is a verb, a noun, an adjective, an adverb, etc. This narrows down the possible meanings of the word to one part of speech. However, this may be insufficient. In a sentence that many birds *migrate* twice yearly, the reader can determine the word is a verb, and that it probably does not mean eat or drink; but it could mean travel, mate, lay eggs, hatch, or molt.

Some words can have a number of different meanings depending on how they are used. For example, the word *fly* has a different meaning in each of the following sentences:

- "His trousers have a fly on them."
- "He swatted the fly on his trousers."
- "Those are some fly trousers."
- "They went fly fishing."
- "She hates to fly."
- "If humans were meant to fly, they would have wings."

As strategies, readers can try substituting a familiar word for an unfamiliar one and see whether it makes sense in the sentence. They can also identify other words in a sentence, offering clues to an unfamiliar word's meaning.

Identifying a Writer's Purpose and Tone

Authors may have many purposes for writing a specific text. Their purposes may be to try and convince readers to agree with their position on a subject, to impart information, or to entertain. Other writers are motivated to write from a desire to express their own feelings. Authors' purposes are their reasons for writing something. A single author may have one overriding purpose for writing or multiple reasons. An author may explicitly state their intention in the text, or the reader may need to infer that intention. Those who read reflectively benefit from identifying the purpose because it enables them to analyze information in the text. By knowing why the author wrote the text, readers can glean ideas for how to approach it. The following is a list of questions readers can ask in order to discern an author's purpose for writing a text:

- From the title of the text, why do you think the author wrote it?
- Was the purpose of the text to provide information to readers?
- Did the author want to describe an event, issue, or individual?
- Was it written to express emotions and thoughts?
- Did the author want to convince readers to consider a particular issue?
- Was the author primarily motivated to write the text to entertain?
- Why do you think the author wrote this text from a certain point of view?
- What is your response to the text as a reader?
- Did the author state their purpose for writing it?

Students should read to interpret information rather than simply content themselves with the basic role as a text consumer. Being able to identify an author's purpose efficiently improves reading comprehension, develops critical thinking, and makes students more likely to consider issues in depth before accepting writers' viewpoints. Authors of fiction frequently write to entertain readers. Another purpose for writing fiction is making a political statement; for example, Jonathan Swift wrote "A Modest Proposal" (1729) as a political satire. Another purpose for writing fiction as well as nonfiction is to persuade readers to take some action or further a particular cause. Fiction authors and poets both frequently write to evoke certain moods; for example, Edgar Allan Poe wrote novels, short stories, and poems that evoke moods of gloom, guilt, terror, and dread. Another purpose of poets is evoking certain emotions: love is popular, as in Shakespeare's sonnets and numerous others. In the poem "The Waste Land" (1922), T.S. Eliot evokes society's alienation, disaffection, sterility, and fragmentation.

Authors seldom directly state their purposes in texts. Some students may be confronted with nonfiction texts such as biographies, histories, magazine and newspaper articles, and instruction manuals, among others. To identify the purpose in nonfiction texts, students can ask the following questions:

- Is the author trying to teach something?
- Is the author trying to persuade the reader?
- Is the author imparting factual information only?
- Is this a reliable source?
- Does the author have some kind of hidden agenda?

To apply author purpose in nonfictional passages, students can also analyze sentence structure, word choice, and transitions to answer the aforementioned questions and to make inferences. For example, authors wanting to convince readers to view a topic negatively often choose words with negative connotations.

Narrative Writing

Narrative writing tells a story. The most prominent examples of narrative writing are fictional novels. Here are some examples:

- Mark Twain's *The Adventures of Tom Sawyer* and *The Adventures of Huckleberry Finn*
- Victor Hugo's *Les Misérables*
- Charles Dickens' *Great Expectations, David Copperfield,* and *A Tale of Two Cities*

- Jane Austen's *Northanger Abbey*, *Mansfield Park*, *Pride and Prejudice*, *Sense and Sensibility*, and *Emma*
- Toni Morrison's Beloved, *The Bluest Eye*, and *Song of Solomon*
- Gabriel García Márquez's *One Hundred Years of Solitude* and *Love in the Time of Cholera*

Some nonfiction works are also written in narrative form. For example, some authors choose a narrative style to convey factual information about a topic, such as a specific animal, country, geographic region, and scientific or natural phenomenon.

Since narrative is the type of writing that tells a story, it must be told by someone, who is the narrator. The narrator may be a fictional character telling the story from their own viewpoint. This narrator uses the first person (*I, me, my, mine, we, us, our*, and *ours*). The narrator may simply be the author; for example, when Louisa May Alcott writes "dear reader" in *Little Women*, she (the author) addresses us as readers. In this case, the novel is typically told in third person, referring to the characters as he, she, they, or them. Another more common technique is the omniscient narrator; i.e. the story is told by an unidentified individual who sees and knows everything about the events and characters—not only their externalized actions, but also their internalized feelings and thoughts. Second person, i.e. writing the story by addressing readers as "you" throughout, is less frequently used.

Expository Writing

Expository writing is also known as informational writing. Its purpose is not to tell a story as in narrative writing, to paint a picture as in descriptive writing, or to persuade readers to agree with something as in argumentative writing. Rather, its point is to communicate information to the reader. As such, the point of view of the author will necessarily be more objective. Whereas other types of writing appeal to the reader's emotions, appeal to the reader's reason by using logic, or use subjective descriptions to sway the reader's opinion or thinking, expository writing seeks to simply to provide facts, evidence, observations, and objective descriptions of the subject matter. Some examples of expository writing include research reports, journal articles, articles and books about historical events or periods, academic subject textbooks, news articles and other factual journalistic reports, essays, how-to articles, and user instruction manuals.

Technical Writing

Technical writing is similar to expository writing in that it is factual, objective, and intended to provide information to the reader. Indeed, it may even be considered a subcategory of expository writing. However, technical writing differs from expository writing in that (1) it is specific to a particular field, discipline, or subject; and (2) it uses the specific technical terminology that belongs only to that area. Writing that uses technical terms is intended only for an audience familiar with those terms. A primary example of technical writing today is writing related to computer programming and use.

Persuasive Writing

Persuasive writing is intended to persuade the reader to agree with the author's position. It is also known as argumentative writing. Some writers may be responding to other writers' arguments, in which case they make reference to those authors or text and then disagree with them. However, another common technique is for the author to anticipate opposing viewpoints in general, both from other authors and from the author's own readers. The author brings up these opposing viewpoints, and then refutes them before they can even be raised, strengthening the author's argument. Writers persuade readers by appealing to the readers' reason and emotion, as well as to their own character and credibility. Aristotle called these appeals *logos*, *pathos*, and *ethos*, respectively.

An Author's Attitude as Revealed in the Tone of a Passage or the Language Used

Some question stems will ask about the author's attitude toward a certain person or idea. While it may seem impossible to know exactly what the author felt toward their subject, there are clues to indicate the emotion, or lack thereof, of the author. Clues like word choice or style will alert readers to the author's attitude. Some possible words that name the author's attitude are listed below:

- Admiring
- Angry
- Critical
- Defensive
- Enthusiastic
- Humorous
- Moralizing
- Neutral
- Objective
- Patriotic
- Persuasive
- Playful
- Sentimental
- Serious
- Supportive
- Sympathetic
- Unsupportive

An author's tone is the author's attitude toward their subject and is usually indicated by word choice. If an author's attitude toward their subject is one of disdain, the author will show the subject in a negative light, using deflating words or words that are negatively-charged. If an author's attitude toward their subject is one of praise, the author will use agreeable words and show the subject in a positive light. If an author takes a neutral tone towards their subject, their words will be neutral as well, and they probably will show all sides of their subject, not just the negative or positive side.

Style is another indication of the author's attitude and includes aspects such as sentence structure, type of language, and formatting. Sentence structure is how a sentence is put together. Sometimes, short, choppy sentences will indicate a certain tone given the surrounding context, while longer sentences may serve to create a buffer to avoid being too harsh, or may be used to explain additional information. Style may also include formal or informal language. Using formal language to talk about a subject may indicate a level of respect. Using informal language may be used to create an atmosphere of friendliness or familiarity with a subject. Again, it depends on the surrounding context whether or not language is used in a negative or positive way. Style may also include formatting, such as determining the length of paragraphs or figuring out how to address the reader at the very beginning of the text.

Distinguishing between Fact and Opinion

Facts and Opinions

A **fact** is a statement that is true empirically or an event that has actually occurred in reality, and can be proven or supported by evidence; it is generally objective. In contrast, an **opinion** is subjective, representing something that someone believes rather than something that exists in the absolute. People's individual understandings, feelings, and perspectives contribute to variations in opinion. Although facts are typically objective in nature, in some instances, a statement of fact may be both factual and yet also subjective. For example, emotions are individual subjective experiences. If an individual says that they feel happy or sad, the feeling is subjective, but the statement is factual; hence, it is a subjective fact. In contrast, if one person tells another that the other is feeling happy or sad—whether this is true or not— that is an assumption or an opinion.

Biases

Biases usually occur when someone allows their personal preferences or ideologies to interfere with what should be an objective decision. In personal situations, someone is biased towards someone if they favor them in an unfair way. In academic writing, being biased in your sources means leaving out objective information that would turn the argument one way or the other. The evidence of bias in academic writing makes the text less credible, so be sure to present all viewpoints when writing, not just your own, so to avoid coming off as biased. Being objective when presenting information or dealing with people usually allows the author to gain more credibility.

Stereotypes

Stereotypes are preconceived notions that place a particular rule or characteristics on an entire group of people. Stereotypes are usually offensive to the group they refer to or to allies of that group, and often have negative connotations. The reinforcement of stereotypes isn't always obvious. Sometimes stereotypes can be very subtle and are still widely used in order for people to understand categories within the world. For example, saying that women are more intuitive or nurturing than men is a stereotype, although this is still an assumption used by many in order to understand differences between one another.

Making Logical Inferences

One technique authors often use to make their fictional stories more interesting is not giving away too much information by providing hints and descriptions. It is then up to the reader to draw a conclusion about the author's meaning by connecting textual clues with the reader's own pre-existing experiences and knowledge. Drawing conclusions is important as a reading strategy for understanding what is occurring in a text. Rather than directly stating who, what, where, when, or why, authors often describe story elements. Then, readers must draw conclusions to understand significant story components. As they go through a text, readers can think about the setting, characters, plot, problem, and solution; whether the author provided any clues for consideration; and combine any story clues with their existing knowledge and experiences to draw conclusions about what occurs in the text.

Making Predictions

Before and during reading, readers can apply the strategy of making **predictions** about what they think may happen next. For example, what plot and character developments will occur in fiction? What points will the author discuss in nonfiction? Making predictions about portions of text they have not yet read prepares readers mentally, and also gives them a purpose for reading. To inform and make predictions about text, the reader can do the following:

- Consider the title of the text and what it implies
- Look at the cover of the book
- Look at any illustrations or diagrams for additional visual information
- Analyze the structure of the text
- Apply outside experience and knowledge to the text

Readers may adjust their predictions as they read. Reader predictions may or may not come true in text.

Making Inferences

Authors describe settings, characters, characters' emotions, and events. Readers must infer to understand the text fully. Inferring enables readers to figure out meanings of unfamiliar words, make predictions about upcoming text, draw conclusions, and reflect on reading. Readers can infer about text before, during, and after reading. In everyday life, we use sensory information to infer. Readers can do the same with text. When authors do not answer all readers' questions, readers must infer by looking at illustrations, considering characters' behaviors, and asking questions during reading. Taking clues from text and connecting text to prior knowledge help to draw conclusions. Readers can infer word meanings, settings, reasons for occurrences, character emotions, pronoun referents, author messages, and answers to questions unstated in text.

Making **inferences** and drawing conclusions involve skills that are quite similar: both require readers to fill in information the author has omitted. Authors may omit information as a technique for inducing readers to discover the outcomes themselves; or they may consider certain information unimportant; or they may assume their reading audience already knows certain information. To make an inference or draw a conclusion about text, readers should observe all facts and arguments the author has presented and consider what they already know from their own personal experiences. Reading students taking multiple-choice tests that refer to text passages can determine correct and incorrect choices based on the information in the passage. For example, from a text passage describing an individual's signs of anxiety while unloading groceries and nervously clutching their wallet at a grocery store checkout, readers can infer or conclude that the individual may not have enough money to pay for everything.

Summarizing

An important skill is the ability to read a complex text and then reduce its length and complexity by focusing on the key events and details. A **summary** is a shortened version of the original text, written by the reader in their own words. The summary should be shorter than the original text, and it must include the most critical points.

In order to effectively summarize a complex text, it's necessary to understand the original source and identify the major points covered. It may be helpful to outline the original text to get the big picture and avoid getting bogged down in the minor details. For example, a summary wouldn't include a statistic from the original source unless it was the major focus of the text. It is also important for readers to use their own words but still retain the original meaning of the passage. The key to a good summary is emphasizing the main idea without changing the focus of the original information.

Complex texts will likely be more difficult to summarize. Readers must evaluate all points from the original source, filter out the unnecessary details, and maintain only the essential ideas. The summary often mirrors the original text's organizational structure. For example, in a problem-solution text structure, the author typically presents readers with a problem and then develops solutions through the course of the text. An effective summary would likely retain this general structure, rephrasing the problem and then reporting the most useful or plausible solutions.

Paraphrasing is somewhat similar to summarizing. It calls for the reader to take a small part of the passage and list or describe its main points. Paraphrasing is more than rewording the original passage, though. As with summary, a paraphrase should be written in the reader's own words, while still retaining the meaning of the original source. The main difference between summarizing and paraphrasing is that a summary would be appropriate for a much larger text, while paraphrase might focus on just a few lines of text. Effective paraphrasing will indicate an understanding of the original source, yet still help the reader expand on their interpretation. A paraphrase should neither add new information nor remove essential facts that change the meaning of the source.

HESI Reading Practice Questions

Questions 1 and 2 are based off the following passage:

Rehabilitation, rather than punitive justice, is becoming much more popular in prisons around the world. Prisons in America, especially, where the recidivism rate is 67 percent, would benefit from mimicking prison tactics in Norway, which has a recidivism rate of only 20 percent. In Norway, the idea is that a rehabilitated prisoner is much less likely to offend than one harshly punished. Rehabilitation includes proper treatment for substance abuse, psychotherapy, health and dental care, and education programs.

1. Which of the following best captures the author's purpose?
   a. To show the audience one of the effects of criminal rehabilitation by comparison
   b. To persuade the audience to donate to American prisons for education programs
   c. To convince the audience of the harsh conditions of American prisons
   d. To inform the audience of the incredibly lax system of Norwegian prisons

2. Which of the following describes the word *recidivism* as it is used in the passage?
   a. The lack of violence in the prison system.
   b. The opportunity of inmates to receive therapy in prison.
   c. The event of a prisoner escaping the compound.
   d. The likelihood of a convicted criminal to reoffend.

Questions 3–5 are based off the following passage from Virginia Woolf's Mrs. Dalloway:

What a lark! What a plunge! For so it had always seemed to her, when, with a little squeak of the hinges, which she could hear now, she had burst open the French windows and plunged at Bourton into the open air. How fresh, how calm, stiller than this of course, the air was in the early morning; like the flap of a wave; the kiss of a wave; chill and sharp and yet (for a girl of eighteen as she then was) solemn, feeling as she did, standing there at the open window, that something awful was about to happen; looking at the flowers, at the trees with the smoke winding off them and the rooks rising, falling; standing and looking until Peter Walsh said, "Musing among the vegetables?"—was that it?—"I prefer men to cauliflowers"—was that it? He must have said it at breakfast one morning when she had gone out on to the terrace—Peter Walsh. He would be back from India one of these days, June or July, she forgot which, for his letters were awfully dull; it was his sayings one remembered; his eyes, his pocket-knife, his smile, his grumpiness and, when millions of things had utterly vanished—how strange it was!—a few sayings like this about cabbages.

3. The passage is reflective of which of the following types of writing?
   a. Persuasive
   b. Expository
   c. Technical
   d. Narrative

4. What was the narrator feeling right before Peter Walsh's voice distracted her?
    a. A spark of excitement for the morning
    b. Anger at the larks
    c. A sense of foreboding
    d. Confusion at the weather

5. What is the main point of the passage?
    a. To present the events leading up to a party
    b. To show the audience that the narrator is resentful towards Peter
    c. To introduce Peter Walsh back into the narrator's memory
    d. To reveal what mornings are like in the narrator's life

Question 6 is based on the following passage from The Federalist No. 78 *by Alexander Hamilton:*

According to the plan of the convention, all judges who may be appointed by the United States are to hold their offices *during good behavior,* which is conformable to the most approved of the State constitutions and among the rest, to that of this State. Its propriety having been drawn into question by the adversaries of that plan, is no light symptom of the rage for objection, which disorders their imaginations and judgments. The standard of good behavior for the continuance in office of the judicial magistracy, is certainly one of the most valuable of the modern improvements in the practice of government. In a monarchy, it is an excellent barrier to the despotism of the prince; in a republic, it is a no less excellent barrier to the encroachments and oppressions of the representative body. And it is the best expedient that can be devised in any government, to secure a steady, upright, and impartial administration of the laws.

6. What is Hamilton's point in this excerpt?
    a. To show the audience that despotism within a monarchy is no longer the standard practice in the states
    b. To convince the audience that judges holding their positions based on good behavior is a practical way to avoid corruption
    c. To persuade the audience that having good behavior should be the primary characteristic of a person in a government body and their voting habits should reflect this
    d. To convey the position that judges who serve for a lifetime will not be perfect, and therefore we must forgive them for their bad behavior when it arises

Questions 7–9 are based on the passage from Many Marriages *by Sherwood Anderson:*

There was a man named Webster who lived in a town of twenty-five thousand people in the state of Wisconsin. He had a wife named Mary and a daughter named Jane and he was himself a fairly prosperous manufacturer of washing machines. When the thing happened of which I am about to write, he was thirty-seven or thirty-eight years old and his one child, the daughter, was seventeen. Of the details of his life up to the time a certain revolution happened within him it will be unnecessary to speak. He was however a rather quiet man inclined to have dreams which he tried to crush out of himself in order that he function as a washing machine manufacturer; and no doubt, at odd moments, when he was on a train going some place or perhaps on Sunday afternoons in the summer when he went alone to the deserted office of the factory and sat several hours looking out at a window and along a railroad track, he gave way to dreams.

7. What does the author mean by the following sentence?

   "Of the details of his life up to the time a certain revolution happened within him it will be unnecessary to speak."

   a. The details of his external life don't matter; only the details of his internal life matter.
   b. Whatever happened in his life before he had a certain internal change is irrelevant.
   c. He had a traumatic experience earlier in his life that rendered it impossible for him to speak.
   d. Before the revolution, he was a lighthearted man who always wished to speak to others no matter who they were.

8. From what Point Of View is this narrative told?
   a. First person limited
   b. First person omniscient
   c. Second person
   d. Third person

9. What did Webster do for a living?
   a. Washing machine manufacturer
   b. Train operator
   c. Leader of the revolution
   d. Stay-at-home husband

Questions 10–12 are based on the following passage from the biography Queen Victoria *by E. Gordon Browne, M.A.:*

> The old castle soon proved to be too small for the family, and in September 1853 the foundation-stone of a new house was laid. After the ceremony, the workmen were entertained at dinner, which was followed by Highland games and dancing in the ballroom.
>
> Two years later, they entered the new castle, which the Queen described as "charming; the rooms delightful; the furniture, papers, everything perfection."
>
> The Prince was untiring in planning improvements, and in 1856 the Queen wrote: "Every year my heart becomes more fixed in this dear Paradise, and so much more so now, that *all* has become my dearest Albert's *own* creation, own work, own building, own laying out as at Osborne; and his great taste, and the impress of his dear hand, have been stamped everywhere. He was very busy today, settling and arranging many things for next year."

10. This excerpt is considered which of the following?
    a. Primary source
    b. Secondary source
    c. Tertiary source
    d. None of these

11. How many years did it take for the new castle to be built?
    a. One year
    b. Two years
    c. Three years
    d. Four years

12. What does the word *impress* mean in the third paragraph?
   a. To affect strongly in feeling
   b. To urge something to be done
   c. To impose a certain quality upon
   d. To press a thing onto something else

Questions 13–15 are based on the following passage from The Life, Crime, and Capture of John Wilkes Booth *by George Alfred Townsend:*

> Having completed these preparations, Mr. Booth entered the theater by the stage door; summoned one of the scene shifters, Mr. John Spangler, emerged through the same door with that individual, leaving the door open, and left the mare in his hands to be held until he (Booth) should return. Booth who was even more fashionably and richly dressed than usual, walked thence around to the front of the theater, and went in. Ascending to the dress circle, he stood for a little time gazing around upon the audience and occasionally upon the stage in his usual graceful manner. He was subsequently observed by Mr. Ford, the proprietor of the theater, to be slowly elbowing his way through the crowd that packed the rear of the dress circle toward the right side, at the extremity of which was the box where Mr. and Mrs. Lincoln and their companions were seated. Mr. Ford casually noticed this as a slightly extraordinary symptom of interest on the part of an actor so familiar with the routine of the theater and the play.

13. How is the above passage organized?
   a. Chronological
   b. Cause and effect
   c. Problem to solution
   d. Main idea with supporting details

14. Based on your knowledge of history, what is about to happen?
   a. An asteroid is about to hit the earth.
   b. The best opera of all times is about to premiere.
   c. A playhouse is about to be burned to the ground.
   d. A president is about to be assassinated.

15. What does the author mean by the last two sentences?
   a. Mr. Ford was suspicious of Booth and assumed he was making his way to Mr. Lincoln's box.
   b. Mr. Ford assumed Booth's movement throughout the theater was due to being familiar with the theater.
   c. Mr. Ford thought that Booth was making his way to the theater lounge to find his companions.
   d. Mr. Ford thought that Booth was elbowing his way to the dressing room to get ready for the play.

Questions 16–20 are based on the following passage from The Story of Germ Life *by Herbert William Conn:*

> When we study more carefully the effect upon the milk of the different species of bacteria found in the dairy, we find that there is a great variety of changes which they produce when they are allowed to grow in milk. The dairyman experiences many troubles with his milk. It sometimes curdles without becoming acid. Sometimes it becomes bitter, or acquires an unpleasant "tainted" taste, or, again, a "soapy" taste. Occasionally a dairyman finds his milk becoming slimy, instead of souring and curdling in the normal fashion. At such times, after a number of hours, the milk

becomes so slimy that it can be drawn into long threads. Such an infection proves very troublesome, for many a time it persists in spite of all attempts made to remedy it. Again, in other cases the milk will turn blue, acquiring about the time it becomes sour a beautiful sky-blue colour. Or it may become red, or occasionally yellow. All of these troubles the dairyman owes to the presence in his milk of unusual species of bacteria which grow there abundantly.

16. What is the author's purpose in writing this passage?
   a. To show the readers that dairymen have difficult jobs
   b. To show the readers different ways their milk might go bad
   c. To show some of the different effects of milk on bacteria
   d. To show some of the different effects of bacteria on milk

17. What is the tone of this passage?
   a. Excitement
   b. Anger
   c. Neutral
   d. Sorrowful

18. Which of the following reactions does NOT occur in the above passage when bacteria infect the milk?
   a. It can have a soapy taste.
   b. The milk will turn black.
   c. It can become slimy.
   d. The milk will turn blue.

19. What is the meaning of "curdle" as depicted in the following sentence?
"Occasionally a dairyman finds his milk becoming slimy, instead of souring and curdling in the normal fashion."
   a. Lumpy
   b. Greasy
   c. Oily
   d. Slippery

20. Why, according to the passage, does an infection with slimy threads prove very troublesome?
   a. Because it is impossible to get rid of.
   b. Because it can make the milk-drinker sick.
   c. Because it turns the milk a blue color.
   d. Because it makes the milk taste bad.

Questions 21–24 are based on the following passage from Oregon, Washington, and Alaska. Sights and Scenes for the Tourist, *written by E.L. Lomax in 1890:*

Portland is a very beautiful city of 60,000 inhabitants, and situated on the Willamette river twelve miles from its junction with the Columbia. It is perhaps true of many of the growing cities of the West, that they do not offer the same social advantages as the older cities of the East. But this is principally the case as to what may be called boom cities, where the larger part of the population is of that floating class which follows in the line of temporary growth for the purposes of speculation, and in no sense applies to those centers of trade whose prosperity is based on the solid foundation of legitimate business. As the metropolis of a vast section of country, having broad agricultural valleys filled with improved farms, surrounded by mountains rich in mineral wealth, and boundless forests of as fine timber as the world produces, the cause of Portland's growth and prosperity is the trade which it has as the center of collection and distribution of this great wealth of natural resources, and it has attracted, not the boomer and speculator, who find their profits in the wild excitement of the boom, but the merchant, manufacturer, and investor, who seek the surer if slower channels of legitimate business and investment. These have come from the East, most of them within the last few years. They came as seeking a better and wider field to engage in the same occupations they had followed in their Eastern homes, and bringing with them all the love of polite life which they had acquired there, have established here a new society, equaling in all respects that which they left behind. Here are as fine churches, as complete a system of schools, as fine residences, as great a love of music and art, as can be found at any city of the East of equal size.

21. What is a characteristic of a "boom city," as indicated by the passage?
    a. A city that is built on solid business foundation of mineral wealth and farming
    b. An area of land on the west coast that quickly becomes populated by residents from the east coast
    c. A city that, due to the hot weather and dry climate, catches fire frequently, resulting in a devastating population drop
    d. A city whose population is made up of people who seek quick fortunes rather than building a solid business foundation

22. The author would classify Portland as which of the following?
    a. A boom city
    b. A city on the east coast
    c. An industrial city
    d. A city of legitimate business

23. What type of passage is this?
    a. A business proposition
    b. A travel guide
    c. A journal entry
    d. A scholarly article

24. What does the word *metropolis* mean in the middle of the passage?
    a. Farm
    b. Country
    c. City
    d. Valley

Questions 25–26 are based on the excerpt from The Golden Bough *by Sir James George Frazer:*

> The other of the minor deities at Nemi was Virbius. Legend had it that Virbius was the young Greek hero Hippolytus, chaste and fair, who learned the art of venery from the centaur Chiron, and spent all his days in the greenwood chasing wild beasts with the virgin huntress Artemis (the Greek counterpart of Diana) for his only comrade.

25. Based on a prior knowledge of literature, the reader can infer this passage is taken from which of the following?
    a. A eulogy
    b. A myth
    c. A historical document
    d. A technical document

26. What is the meaning of the word *comrade* as the last word in the passage?
    a. Friend
    b. Enemy
    c. Brother
    d. Pet

Questions 27–29 are based on Poems by Alexander Pushkin *by Ivan Panin:*

> I do not believe there are as many as five examples of deviation from the literalness of the text. Once only, I believe, have I transposed two lines for convenience of translation; the other deviations are (*if* they are such) a substitution of an *and* for a comma in order to make now and then the reading of a line musical. With these exceptions, I have sacrificed *everything* to faithfulness of rendering. My object was to make Pushkin himself, without a prompter, speak to English readers. To make him thus speak in a foreign tongue was indeed to place him at a disadvantage; and music and rhythm and harmony are indeed fine things, but truth is finer still. I wished to present not what Pushkin would have said, or should have said, if he had written in English, but what he does say in Russian. That, stripped from all ornament of his wonderful melody and grace of form, as he is in a translation, he still, even in the hard English tongue, soothes and stirs, is in itself a sign that through the individual soul of Pushkin sings that universal soul whose strains appeal forever to man, in whatever clime, under whatever sky.

27. What is meant by the last sentence of the passage?
    a. That the artistic beauty of Pushkin's poetry runs so deep that it is retained in translations to any language
    b. That the artistic beauty of Pushkin's poetry is lost in the hard English tone
    c. That Pushkin's poetry should not be translated because it strips it of its artistic beauty and meaning
    d. That Pushkin's poetry is written in a universal language, so it does not need to be translated

28. Where would you most likely find this passage in a text?
    a. Appendix
    b. Table of contents
    c. First chapter
    d. Preface

29. According to the author, what is the most important aim of translation work?
    a. To retain the beauty of the work.
    b. To retain the truth of the work.
    c. To retain the melody of the work.
    d. To retain the form of the work.

Questions 30–33 are based on the following passage from Variation of Animals and Plants *by Charles Darwin:*

> Peach (*Amygdalus persica*)—In the last chapter I gave two cases of a peach-almond and a double-flowered almond which suddenly produced fruit closely resembling true peaches. I have also given many cases of peach-trees producing buds, which, when developed into branches, have yielded nectarines. We have seen that no less than six named and several unnamed varieties of the peach have thus produced several varieties of nectarine. I have shown that it is highly improbable that all these peach-trees, some of which are old varieties, and have been propagated by the million, are hybrids from the peach and nectarine, and that it is opposed to all analogy to attribute the occasional production of nectarines on peach-trees to the direct action of pollen from some neighbouring nectarine-tree. Several of the cases are highly remarkable, because, firstly, the fruit thus produced has sometimes been in part a nectarine and in part a peach; secondly, because nectarines thus suddenly produced have reproduced themselves by seed; and thirdly, because nectarines are produced from peach-trees from seed as well as from buds. The seed of the nectarine, on the other hand, occasionally produces peaches; and we have seen in one instance that a nectarine-tree yielded peaches by bud-variation. As the peach is certainly the oldest or primary variety, the production of peaches from nectarines, either by seeds or buds, may perhaps be considered as a case of reversion. Certain trees have also been described as indifferently bearing peaches or nectarines, and this may be considered as bud-variation carried to an extreme degree.

30. Which of the following statements is NOT a detail from the passage?
    a. At least six named varieties of the peach have produced several varieties of nectarine.
    b. It is not probable that all of the peach trees mentioned are hybrids from the peach and nectarine.
    c. An unremarkable case is the fact that nectarines are produced from peach trees from seeds as well as from buds.
    d. The production of peaches from nectarines might be considered a case of reversion.

31. What is the meaning of the word *propagated* in this passage?
    a. Multiplied
    b. Diminished
    c. Watered
    d. Uprooted

32. What is the author's tone in this passage?
    a. Enthusiastic
    b. Objective
    c. Critical
    d. Desperate

33. Which of the following is an accurate paraphrasing of the following sentence?

Certain trees have also been described as indifferently bearing peaches or nectarines, and this may be considered as bud-variation carried to an extreme degree.

a. Some trees are described as bearing peaches, and some trees have been described as bearing nectarines, but individually, the buds are extreme examples of variation.

b. One way in which bud variation is said to be carried to an extreme degree is when specific trees have been shown to casually produce peaches or nectarines.

c. Certain trees are indifferent to bud variation, as recently shown in the trees that produce both peaches and nectarines in the same season.

d. Nectarines and peaches are known to have cross-variation in their buds, which indifferently bear other sorts of fruit to an extreme degree.

Questions 34–39 are based on the following passage from A Christmas Carol *by Charles Dickens:*

Meanwhile the fog and darkness thickened so, that people ran about with flaring links, proffering their services to go before horses in carriages, and conduct them on their way. The ancient tower of a church, whose gruff old bell was always peeping slyly down at Scrooge out of a Gothic window in the wall, became invisible, and struck the hours and quarters in the clouds, with tremulous vibrations afterwards as if its teeth were chattering in its frozen head up there. The cold became intense. In the main street, at the corner of the court, some labourers were repairing the gas-pipes, and had lighted a great fire in a brazier, round which a party of ragged men and boys were gathered: warming their hands and winking their eyes before the blaze in rapture. The water-plug being left in solitude, its overflowings sullenly congealed, and turned to misanthropic ice. The brightness of the shops where holly sprigs and berries crackled in the lamp heat of the windows, made pale faces ruddy as they passed. Poulterers' and grocers' trades became a splendid joke; a glorious pageant, with which it was next to impossible to believe that such dull principles as bargain and sale had anything to do. The Lord Mayor, in the stronghold of the mighty Mansion House, gave orders to his fifty cooks and butlers to keep Christmas as a Lord Mayor's household should; and even the little tailor, whom he had fined five shillings on the previous Monday for being drunk and bloodthirsty in the streets, stirred up to-morrow's pudding in his garret, while his lean wife and the baby sallied out to buy the beef.

34. In the context in which it appears, *congealed* most nearly means which of the following?

a. Burst

b. Loosened

c. Shrank

d. Thickened

35. Which of the following can NOT be inferred from the passage?

a. The season of this narrative is in the wintertime.

b. The majority of the narrative is located in a bustling city street.

c. This passage takes place during the nighttime.

d. The Lord Mayor is a wealthy person within the narrative.

36. According to the passage, which of the following is true about the poulterers and grocers?

a. They were so poor in the quality of their products that customers saw them as a joke.

b. They put on a pageant in the streets every year for Christmas to entice their customers.

c. They did not believe in Christmas, so they refused to participate in the town parade.

d. They set their shops up to be entertaining public spectacles rather than a dull trade exchange.

37. What is the meaning of the word *proffering* in this passage?
    a. Giving away
    b. Offering
    c. Bolstering
    d. Teaching

38. What does the author mean by the following sentence?
    The brightness of the shops where holly sprigs and berries crackled in the lamp heat of the windows, made pale faces ruddy as they passed.

    a. When people walked past the shops, their faces turned red because of the lamps in the windows that were also lighting up holly sprigs and berries.
    b. Compared with the holly sprigs and berries and their crackling lamplight, everyone's face looked old when they walked by the shops.
    c. When people walked past the shops, their faces looked cold and blue compared with the warm light of the shops, which were making the holly sprigs and berries glow.
    d. While shop owners were cooking their holly sprigs and berries in the warm glow of the fire, people's faces lit up with excitement as they passed.

39. Which statement is NOT a detail from the passage?
    a. There was a pageant in the town square.
    b. There was an old clock that tolled behind the clouds.
    c. There were workers that were repairing gas pipes.
    d. The tailor's wife went out to buy beef.

Questions 40–45 are based on the following passage from the novel Frankenstein *by Mary Wollstonecraft Shelley:*

I trembled excessively; I could not endure to think of, and far less to allude to, the occurrences of the preceding night. I walked with a quick pace, and we soon arrived at my college. I then reflected, and the thought made me shiver, that the creature whom I had left in my apartment might still be there, alive, and walking about. I dreaded to behold this monster; but I feared still more that Henry should see him. Entreating him, therefore, to remain a few minutes at the bottom of the stairs, I darted up towards my own room. My hand was already on the lock of the door before I recollected myself. I then paused; and a cold shivering came over me. I threw the door forcibly open, as children are accustomed to do when they expect a spectre to stand in waiting for them on the other side; but nothing appeared. I stepped fearfully in: the apartment was empty; and my bed-room was also freed from its hideous guest. I could hardly believe that so great a good fortune could have befallen me; but when I became assured that my enemy had indeed fled, I clapped my hands for joy, and ran down to Clerval.

40. What is the meaning of the word *entreating* in the passage?
    a. To yell or demand
    b. To criticize
    c. To ask or beg
    d. To speak softly to

41. Which statement is NOT a detail from the passage?
    a. The speaker trembles when thinking about the occurrences the night before.
    b. The speaker throws his own door open in a flurry.
    c. The speaker claps his hands for joy and runs down to his friend.
    d. The speaker sees a ghost in his home when he opens the door.

42. Which of the following sentences best summarizes the passage?
    a. The speaker meets his friend at an abandoned building where they attempt to hunt a creature that terrorized them the night before.
    b. The speaker and a friend arrive at the apartment where, to the speaker's relief, a terrifying creature from the night before appears to have left the space.
    c. The speaker is angry at his friend for letting loose a terrifying creature in his house, only to find the creature gone.
    d. The speaker is eager to show his friend a terrifying creature locked inside his apartment, only to find that the creature has disappeared from the apartment.

43. In the context of the passage, *behold* means which of the following?
    a. Touch
    b. Hold
    c. Witness
    d. Hurt

44. Which of the following is an accurate paraphrasing of the sentence below?
    I could hardly believe that so great a good fortune could have befallen me; but when I became assured that my enemy had indeed fled, I clapped my hands for joy, and ran down to Clerval.

    a. At first, I thought I had great fortune; however, when I came to my senses about Clerval being my enemy, I resolved to clap my hands for joy and run down to him.
    b. When I realized that the enemy had fled, I knew I had run out of great fortune; try as I might, I could not run down to Clerval clapping my hands in joy.
    c. I had great fortune that had befallen me up until the point when I realized my enemy had fled; then I clapped my hands in happiness and ran down to Clerval.
    d. Even though, at first, I couldn't believe my luck, when I was sure the creature was nowhere to be seen, I happily clapped and ran down to Clerval.

45. Which of the following can NOT be inferred from the passage?
    a. The creature mentioned is Frankenstein.
    b. Henry does not know of the creature's existence.
    c. The speaker is terrified of the creature.
    d. The speaker is attending a college.

Questions 46–50 are based on the following passage from the book On the Trail *by Lina Beard and Adelia Belle Beard:*

> For any journey, by rail or by boat, one has a general idea of the direction to be taken, the character of the land or water to be crossed, and of what one will find at the end. So it should be in striking the trail. Learn all you can about the path you are to follow. Whether it is plain or obscure, wet or dry; where it leads; and its length, measured more by time than by actual miles. A smooth, even trail of five miles will not consume the time and strength that must be expended

upon a trail of half that length which leads over uneven ground, varied by bogs and obstructed by rocks and fallen trees, or a trail that is all up-hill climbing. If you are a novice and accustomed to walking only over smooth and level ground, you must allow more time for covering the distance than an experienced person would require and must count upon the expenditure of more strength, because your feet are not trained to the wilderness paths with their pitfalls and traps for the unwary, and every nerve and muscle will be strained to secure a safe foothold amid the tangled roots, on the slippery, moss-covered logs, over precipitous rocks that lie in your path. It will take time to pick your way over boggy places where the water oozes up through the thin, loamy soil as through a sponge; and experience alone will teach you which hummock of grass or moss will make a safe stepping-place and will not sink beneath your weight and soak your feet with hidden water. Do not scorn to learn all you can about the trail you are to take . . . It is not that you hesitate to encounter difficulties, but that you may prepare for them. In unknown regions take a responsible guide with you, unless the trail is short, easily followed, and a frequented one. Do not go alone through lonely places; and, being on the trail, keep it and try no explorations of your own, at least not until you are quite familiar with the country and the ways of the wild.

46. What is the meaning of the word *novice* in this passage?
    a. Expert
    b. Beginner
    c. Child
    d. Adult

47. What does the author say about unknown regions?
    a. You should try and explore unknown regions to learn the land better.
    b. Unless the trail is short or frequented, you should take a responsible guide with you.
    c. All unknown regions will contain pitfalls, traps, and boggy places.
    d. It's better to travel unknown regions by rail than by foot.

48. Which statement is NOT a detail from the passage?
    a. Learning about the trail beforehand is imperative.
    b. Time will differ depending on the land.
    c. Once you are familiar with the outdoors, you can go places on your own.
    d. Be careful of wild animals on the trail you are on.

49. What type of passage is this?
    a. Descriptive
    b. Persuasive
    c. Narrative
    d. Informative

50. Which of the following is the closest definition of the word *precipitous*?
    a. Extremely slippery
    b. Dangerously steep
    c. Highly sharp
    d. Unusually pliable

The following is entitled Architecture and Democracy *by Claude Bragdon. The next five questions are based on the following passage.*

The world war represents not the triumph, but the birth of democracy. The true ideal of democracy—the rule of a people by the *demos*, or group soul—is a thing unrealized. How then is it possible to consider or discuss an architecture of democracy—the shadow of a shade? It is not possible to do so with any degree of finality, but by an intention of consciousness upon this juxtaposition of ideas—architecture and democracy—signs of the times may yield new meanings, relations may emerge between things apparently unrelated, and the future, always existent in every present moment, may be evoked by that strange magic which resides in the human mind.

Architecture, at its worst as at its best, reflects always a true image of the thing that produced it; a building is revealing even though it is false, just as the face of a liar tells the thing his words endeavor to conceal. This being so, let us make such architecture as is ours declare to us our true estate.

The architecture of the United States, from the period of the Civil War, up to the beginning of the present crisis, everywhere reflects a struggle to be free of a vicious and depraved form of feudalism, grown strong under the very ægis of democracy. The qualities that made feudalism endeared and enduring; qualities written in beauty on the cathedral cities of mediaeval Europe—faith, worship, loyalty, magnanimity—were either vanished or banished from this pseudo-democratic, aridly scientific feudalism, leaving an inheritance of strife and tyranny—a strife grown mean, a tyranny grown prudent, but full of sinister power the weight of which we have by no means ceased to feel.

Power, strangely mingled with timidity; ingenuity, frequently misdirected; ugliness, the result of a false ideal of beauty—these in general characterize the architecture of our immediate past; an architecture "without ancestry or hope of posterity," an architecture devoid of coherence or conviction; willing to lie, willing to steal. What impression such a city as Chicago or Pittsburgh might have made upon some denizen of those cathedral-crowned feudal cities of the past we do not know. He would certainly have been amazed at its giant energy, and probably revolted at its grimy dreariness. We are wont to pity the mediaeval man for the dirt he lived in, even while smoke greys our sky and dirt permeates the very air we breathe: we think of castles as grim and cathedrals as dim, but they were beautiful and gay with color compared with the grim, dim canyons of our city streets.

51. Which of the following does the author NOT consider to be a characteristic of modern architecture?
    a. Power, strangely mingled with timidity
    b. Ugliness as a result of the false ideal of beauty
    c. Giant energy with grimy dreariness
    d. Cathedral-crowned grim and dim castles

52. By stating that "Architecture, at its worst as at its best, reflects always a true image of the thing that produced it," the author most likely intends to suggest that:
    a. People always create buildings to look like themselves.
    b. Architecture gets more grim, drab, and depressing as the years go by.
    c. Architecture reflects—in shape, color, and form—the attitude of the society which built it.
    d. Modern architecture is a lot like democracy because it is uniform yet made up of more pieces than your traditional architecture.

53. The author refers to "mediaeval man" in the fourth paragraph in order to:
    a. Make the audience look at feudalism with a sense of nostalgia and desire.
    b. Make the audience feel gratitude for modern comforts such as architecture.
    c. Make the audience realize the irony produced from pitying him.
    d. Make the audience look back at feudalism as a time which was dark and dreary.

54. Based on the discussion in paragraph 3, which of the following would be considered architecture from medieval Europe?
    a. Canyon
    b. Castle
    c. Factory
    d. Skyscraper

55. The author's attitude toward modern architecture can best be characterized as:
    a. Narcissistic
    b. Aggrieved
    c. Virtuous
    d. Sarcastic

Answer Explanations

1. A: The author's purpose is to show the audience one of the effects of criminal rehabilitation by comparison. Choice *B* is incorrect because although it is obvious the author favors rehabilitation, the author never asks for donations from the audience. Choices *C* and *D* are also incorrect. We can infer from the passage that American prisons are probably harsher than Norwegian prisons. However, the best answer that captures the author's purpose is Choice *A*, because we see an effect by the author (recidivism rate of each country) comparing Norwegian and American prisons.

2. D: The likelihood of a convicted criminal to reoffend. The passage explains how a Norwegian prison, due to rehabilitation, has a smaller rate of recidivism. Thus, we can infer that recidivism is probably not a positive attribute. Choices *A* and *B* are both positive attributes—the lack of violence and the opportunity of inmates to receive therapy—so Norway would probably not have a lower rate of these two things. Choice *C* is possible, but it does not make sense in context because the author does not talk about tactics to keep prisoners inside the compound but ways in which to rehabilitate criminals so that they can live as citizens when they get out of prison.

3. D: The passage is reflective of a narrative. A narrative is used to tell a story, as we see the narrator trying to do so in this passage by using memory and dialogue. Choice *A*, persuasive writing, uses rhetorical devices to try to convince the audience of something, and there is no persuasion or argument within this passage. Choice *B*, expository, is a type of writing used to inform the reader. Choice *C*, technical writing, is usually used within business communications and uses technical language to explain procedures or concepts to someone within the same technical field.

4. C: The narrator was feeling a sense of foreboding. The narrator, after feeling excitement for the morning, feels "that something awful was about to happen," which is considered foreboding. The narrator mentions larks and weather in the passage, but there is no proof of anger or confusion at either of them.

5. C: The main point of the passage is to introduce Peter Walsh back into the narrator's memory. Choice *A* is incorrect because, although the novel *Mrs. Dalloway* is about events leading up to a party, the passage does not mention anything about a party. Choice *B* is incorrect; the narrator calls Peter *dull* at one point, but the rest of her memories of him are more positive. Choice *D* is incorrect; although morning is described within the first few sentences of the passage, the passage quickly switches to a description of Peter Walsh and the narrator's memories of him.

6. B: The point is to convince the audience that judges holding their positions based on good behavior is a practical way to avoid corruption.

7. B: The sentence is best taken to mean that whatever happened in his life before he had a certain internal change is irrelevant. Choices *A*, *C*, and *D* use some of the same language as the original passage, like "revolution," "speak," and "details," but they do not capture the meaning of the statement. The narrator was not concerned with the character's life before his epiphany and had no intention of talking about it.

8. B: It is told in first-person omniscient. This is the best guess with the information we have. In the world of the passage, the narrator is first-person because we see them use the "I," but they also know the actions and thoughts of the protagonist, a character named "Webster." First-person limited tells their own story, making Choice *A* incorrect. Choice *C* is incorrect; second person uses "you" to tell the story. Third

67

person uses "them," "they," etc., and would not fall into use of the "I" in the narrative, making Choice *D* incorrect.

9. A: Webster is a washing machine manufacturer. This question assesses reading comprehension. We see in the second sentence that Webster "was a fairly prosperous manufacturer of washing machines," making Choice A the correct answer.

10. B: This excerpt is considered a secondary source because it actively interprets primary sources. We see direct quotes from the queen, which would be considered a primary source. But since we see those quotes being interpreted and analyzed, the excerpt becomes a secondary source. Choice *C*, tertiary source, is an index of secondary and primary sources, like an encyclopedia or Wikipedia.

11. B: It took two years for the new castle to be built. The author states this in the first sentence of the second paragraph. In the third year, we see the Prince planning improvements and arranging things for the fourth year.

12. C: In this context, *impress* means to impose a certain quality upon. The sentence states that "the impress of his dear hand [has] been stamped everywhere," regarding the quality of his tastes and creations on the house. Choice *A* is one definition of *impress*, but this definition is used more as a verb than a noun: "She impressed us as a songwriter." Choice *B* is incorrect because it is also used as a verb: "He impressed the need for something to be done." Choice *D* is incorrect because it is part of a physical act: "the businessman impressed his mark upon the envelope." The phrase in the passage is figurative, since the workmen did most of the physical labor, not the Prince.

13. A: The passage presents us with a sequence of events that happens in chronological order. Choice *B* is incorrect. Cause and effect organization would usually explain why something happened or list the effects of something. Choice *C* is incorrect because problem and solution organization would detail a problem and then present a solution to the audience, and there is no solution presented here. Finally, Choice *D* is incorrect. We are entered directly into the narrative without any main idea or any kind of argument being delivered.

14. D: A president is about to be assassinated. The context clues in the passage give hints to what is about to happen. The passage mentions John Wilkes Booth as "Mr. Booth," the man who shot Abraham Lincoln. The passage also mentions a "Mr. Ford," and we know that Lincoln was shot in Ford's theater. Finally, the passage mentions Mr. and Mrs. Lincoln. By adding all these clues up and layering them on our prior knowledge of history, the assassination of President Lincoln by Booth in Ford's theater is probably the next thing that is going to happen.

15. B: Mr. Ford assumed Booth's movement throughout the theater was due to being familiar with the theater. Choice *A* is incorrect; although Booth does eventually make his way to Lincoln's box, Mr. Ford does not make this distinction in this part of the passage. Choice *C* is incorrect; although the passage mentions "companions," it mentions Lincoln's companions rather than Booth's companions. Finally, Choice *D* is incorrect; the passage mentions "dress circle," which means the first level of the theater, but this is different from a "dressing room."

16. D: The passage explains the different ways bacteria can affect milk by detailing the color and taste of different infections. Choices *A* and *B* might be true, but they are not the main purpose of the passage as detailed in the first sentence. Choice *C* is incorrect, since milk does not have an effect on bacteria in this particular passage.

17. C: The tone of this passage is neutral, since it is written in an academic/informative voice. It is important to look at the author's word choice to determine the tone of a passage. We have no indication that the author is excited, angry, or sorrowful at the effects of bacteria on milk, so Choices *A, B,* and *D* are incorrect.

18. B: The milk will turn black is not a reaction mentioned in the passage. The passage does state, however, that the milk may get "soapy," that it can become "slimy," and that it may turn out to be a "beautiful sky-blue colour," making Choices *A, C,* and *D* incorrect.

19. A: In the sentence, we know that the word "curdle" means the opposite of "slimy." The words greasy, oily, and slippery are all very similar to the word slimy, making Choices *B, C,* and *D* incorrect. "Lumpy" means clotted, chunky, or thickened.

20. A: It is troublesome because it is impossible to get rid of. The passage mentions milk turning blue or tasting bad, and milk could possibly even make a milk-drinker sick if it has slimy threads. However, we know for sure that the slimy threads prove troublesome because they can become impossible to get rid of from this sentence: "Such an infection proves very troublesome, for many a time it persists in spite of all attempts made to remedy it."

21. D: A "boom city" is a city whose population is made up of people who seek quick fortunes rather than building a solid business foundation. Choice *A* is a characteristic of Portland but not that of a boom city. Choice *B* is close—a boom city is one that becomes quickly populated, but it is not necessarily always populated by residents from the east coast. Choice *C* is incorrect because a boom city is not one that catches fire frequently, but one made up of people who are looking to make quick fortunes from the resources provided on the land.

22. D: The author would classify Portland as a city of legitimate business. We can see the proof in this sentence: "the cause of Portland's growth and prosperity is the trade which it has as the center of collection and distribution of this great wealth of natural resources, and it has attracted, not the boomer and speculator . . . but the merchant, manufacturer, and investor, who seek the surer if slower channels of legitimate business and investment." Choices *A, B,* and *C* are not mentioned in the passage and are incorrect.

23. B: This passage is part of a travel guide. Our first hint is in the title: *Oregon, Washington, and Alaska. Sights and Scenes for the Tourist.* Although the passage talks about business, there is no proposition included, which makes Choice *A* incorrect. Choice *C* is incorrect because the style of the writing is more informative and formal rather than personal and informal. Choice *D* is incorrect; this could possibly be a scholarly article, but the best choice is that it is a travel guide, due to the title and the details of what the city has to offer at the very end.

24. C: *Metropolis* means city. Portland is described as having agricultural valleys, but it is not solely a "farm" or "valley," making Choices *A* and *D* incorrect. We know from the description of Portland that it is more representative of a city than a countryside or country, making Choice *B* incorrect.

25. B: The passage is taken from a myth. Look for the key words that give away the type of passage this is, such as "deities," "Greek hero," "centaur," and the names of demigods like Artemis. A eulogy is typically a speech given at a funeral, making Choice *A* incorrect. Choices *C* and *D* are incorrect, as "virgin huntresses" and "centaurs" are typically not found in historical or professional documents.

26. A: Based on the context of the passage, we can see that Hippolytus was a friend to Artemis because he "spent all his days in the greenwood chasing wild beasts" with her. The other choices are incorrect.

27. A: The author is saying that the artistic beauty of Pushkin's poetry runs so deep that it is retained even in its translation to the "hard English tongue" or to any language. He says that even though translating the work out of its original Russian form removes its "wonderful melody and grace of form," the poetry is so universal that it will "appeal forever to man, in whatever clime, under whatever sky." This means the author believes Pushkin's poetry is so beautiful that it will appeal to readers all over the world (in different climes (climates) and skies (locations)) and throughout time.

28. D: You would most likely find this in the preface. A preface to a text usually explains what the author has done or aims to do with the work. An appendix is usually found at the end of a text and does not talk about what the author intends to do to the work, making Choice *A* incorrect. A table of contents does not contain prose, but bullet points listing chapters and sections found in the text, making Choice *B* incorrect. Choice *C* is incorrect; the first chapter would include the translated work (here, poetry) and not the author's intentions.

29. B: The most important aim, according to the author, is to retain the truth of the work. The author says that "music and rhythm and harmony are indeed fine things, but truth is finer still," which means that the author stuck to a literal translation instead of changing up any words that might make the English language translation sound better.

30. C: Choice *C* is correct because the word *unremarkable* should be changed to *remarkable* to be consistent with the details of the passage. This question requires close attention to the passage. Choice *A* is incorrect; it can be found where the passage says, "no less than six named and several unnamed varieties of the peach have thus produced several varieties of nectarine." Choice *B* is incorrect; it can be found where the passage says, "it is highly improbable that all these peach-trees . . . are hybrids from the peach and nectarine." Choice *D* is incorrect because we see in the passage that "the production of peaches from nectarines, either by seeds or buds, may perhaps be considered as a case of reversion."

31. A: Choice *A* is correct because the word *multiplied* is synonymous with the word *propagated*. Choice *B* is incorrect because *diminished* means "to decrease or recede" and is the opposite of *propagated*. Choice *C* is incorrect; *watered* is close because it pertains to the growth of trees, but it is not exactly the same thing as *propagated*. Finally, Choice *D* is incorrect; *uprooted* could also pertain to trees, but this answer is incorrect.

32. B: Choice *B* is correct because an objective tone means that the author is open-minded and detached about the subject. Most scientific articles are objective. Choices *A, C,* and *D* are incorrect; the author is not very enthusiastic in the text; the author is not critical but rather interested in the topic; and the author is not desperate in any way here.

33. B: Choice *B* is correct because the meaning holds true even if the words have been switched out or rearranged some. Choice *A* is incorrect because it has trees either bearing peaches or nectarines, and the trees in the original phrase bear both. Choice *C* is incorrect because the statement does not say these trees are "indifferent to bud-variation," but that they have "indifferently [bore] peaches or nectarines." Choice *D* is incorrect; the statement may use some of the same words, but the meaning is skewed in this sentence.

34. D: Choice *D* is correct because we see liquid turning into ice. Choices *A, B,* and *C* are therefore incorrect.

70

35. C: Choice *C* is correct; we cannot infer that the passage takes place during the nighttime. While we do have a statement that says that the darkness thickened, this is the only evidence we have. The darkness could be thickening because it is foggy outside. We don't have enough proof to infer this otherwise. Choice *A* is incorrect; some of the evidence here is that "the cold became intense," and people were decorating their shops with "holly sprigs," a Christmas tradition. It also mentions that it's Christmas time at the end of the passage. Choice *B* is incorrect; we *can* infer that the narrative is located in a bustling city street by the actions in the story. People are running around trying to sell things, the atmosphere is busy, there is a church tolling the hours, etc. The scene switches to the Mayor's house at the end of the passage, but the answer says *majority*, so this is still incorrect. Choice *D* is incorrect; we *can* infer that the Lord Mayor is wealthy—he lives in the "Mansion House" and has fifty cooks.

36. D: Choice *D* is correct because the passage tells us that the poulterers' and grocers' trades were "a glorious pageant, with which it was next to impossible to believe that such dull principles as bargain and sale had anything to do," which means they set up their shops to be entertaining public spectacles to increase sales. Choice *A* is incorrect; although the word *joke* is used, it is meant to be used as a source of amusement rather than something made in poor quality. Choice *B* is incorrect; that they put on a "pageant" is figurative for the public spectacle they made with their shops, not a literal play. Finally, Choice *C* is incorrect; this is not mentioned anywhere in the passage.

37. B: Choice *B* is correct because *proffering* means "to offer something." Choice *A*, giving away, is incorrect. Choice *C* is incorrect because *bolstering* means "helping" or "maintaining." Choice *D*, teaching, is incorrect because it doesn't make sense in the context of the passage.

38. A: Choice *A* is correct. *Ruddy* means "red," so we can deduce that the phrase *made pale faces ruddy* means that the shops made people's faces look red. This is a descriptive sentence, so a careful reading of what's going on is imperative. Choices *B*, *C*, and *D*, although they may contain components of the original meaning, are incorrect.

39. A: Choice *A* is correct because the "pageant" mentioned is only a metaphor to describe the trade going on, and not an actual pageant. Choices *B*, *C*, and *D* are incorrect because they can be found in the passage.

40. C: Choice *C* is correct because the meaning of the word *entreating* is "to ask or beg." The speaker is asking the friend to "remain a few minutes at the bottom of the stairs." Therefore, Choices *A*, *B*, and *D* are incorrect.

41. D: Choice *D* is correct because it is not a detail in the passage, although it is close to a detail in the passage. The passage says that the speaker threw the door open as a child would when they expected to see a spectre, but this doesn't mean that the speaker sees a spectre himself. Choices *A*, *B*, and *C* are incorrect because they can be found as details in the passage.

42. B: Choice *B* is correct. The passage details the speaker and his friend going to the apartment. The speaker, terrified of finding the "creature," realizes that the creature is gone after he barges in through the door. Choice *A* is incorrect because we never see the speaker and the friend trying to hunt anything. Choice *C* is incorrect because we do not have proof that the friend let loose a terrifying creature in the speaker's house. Choice *D* is also incorrect because we have no proof that the speaker is "eager" to show the creature. We see that the speaker is more reluctant to find the creature inside the apartment than eager and does not wish to show any of the friends.

43. C: Choice *C* is correct because the speaker dreaded seeing, or witnessing, the creature in the apartment. Choices *A, B,* and *D* are therefore incorrect.

44. D: Choice *D* is correct because we see the speaker hardly believing his luck, making sure the creature was gone, and then clapping for joy and running to his friend. Choice *A* is incorrect; Clerval is not meant to be the enemy of the speaker in this sentence. Choice *B* is incorrect and is actually the opposite of what the speaker is saying. The speaker *is* in great fortune and *does* clap his hands for joy. Finally, Choice *C* is incorrect; the phrase *up until the point* puts a limitation on the fortune, which is not the intended meaning of the original statement.

45. A: Choice *A* is correct because, although we know from the title of the work that the passage is from *Frankenstein,* we cannot deduce from the passage itself that the creature mentioned is Frankenstein. In fact, the name Frankenstein in the novel is the name of the doctor, or the speaker of the text, and the creature remains unnamed throughout the entirety of the novel. Choice *B* is incorrect because we see that the speaker fears "that Henry should see him." Choice *C* is incorrect; we see the speaker trembling and terrified to "behold" the creature. Choice *D* is incorrect; we do have proof that the speaker is attending college with the sentence, "and we soon arrived at my college."

46. B: Choice *B* is correct. We can use context clues to solve this. The passage states, "if you are a novice and accustomed to walking only over smooth and level ground," which implies that whoever a "novice" is would only be accustomed to smooth ground, not rough ground. An expert would be accustomed to rockier ground than the passage indicates.

47. B: Choice *B* is correct because the sentence states, "In unknown regions take a responsible guide with you, unless the trail is short, easily followed, and a frequented one." Choice *A* is incorrect; the passage does not state that you should try and explore unknown regions. Choice *C* is incorrect; the passage talks about trails that contain pitfalls, traps, and boggy places, but it does not say that *all* unknown regions contain these things. Choice *D* is incorrect; the passage mentions "rail" and "boat" as means of transport at the beginning, but it does not suggest it is better to travel unknown regions by rail.

48. D: Choice *D* is correct because, although it may be real advice an experienced hiker would give to an inexperienced hiker, the question asks about details in the passage, and this is not in the passage. Choice *A* is incorrect; we do see the author encouraging the reader to learn about the trail beforehand: "wet or dry; where it leads; and its length." Choice *B* is also incorrect; we do see the author telling us the time will lengthen with boggy or rugged places opposed to smooth places. Choice *C* is incorrect; at the end of the passage, the author tells us, "do not go alone through lonely places . . . unless you are quite familiar with the country and the ways of the wild."

49. D: Choice *D* is correct because informative passages explain to the readers how to do something; in this case, the author is attempting to explain the fundamentals of camping and hiking. Choice *A* is incorrect because *descriptive* is a type of passage describing a character, event, or place in great detail and imagery. Choice *B* is incorrect because a persuasive passage is an argument that tries to get readers to agree with something. Choice *C* is incorrect because a narrative is a passage that tells a story.

50. B: Choice B is correct because *precipitous* means "dangerously steep." Choices *A, C,* and *D* are therefore incorrect.

51. D: The author does not consider modern architecture to be "cathedral-crowned grim and dim castles." The author is speaking of feudal architecture when they refer to cathedral-crowned cities and castles.

Choices *A, B,* and *C* are all mentioned in the text as characteristics of modern architecture, especially in the cities of Chicago and Pittsburgh.

52. C: Architecture reflects—in shape, color, and form—the attitude of the society which built it. Choice *A* is too specific and is taken too literally. It is not that the architecture represents the builders; it represents the builder's culture. Choice *B* is also incorrect; we do see the words "at its worst as at its best," but the meaning of this is skewed in Choice *B*. Choice *D* is incorrect; the statement does not suggest this analysis.

53. C: The author refers to the "mediaeval man" in order to make the audience realize the irony produced from pitying him. The author says that we pity him for the dirt he lived in; however, we inhale smoke and dirt from our own skies. Choices *A, B,* and *D* are incorrect, as they just miss the mark of the statement.

54. B: The text talks about castles and cathedrals as examples of architecture from medieval Europe. Factories and skyscrapers are considered pre-modern or modern architecture. The term *canyons* is used as a metaphor for city streets, presumably surrounded by tall structures, so Choice *A* is incorrect.

55. B: Considering the strong, negative language used throughout the passage, such as "power, strangely mingled with timidity," "ingenuity, frequently misdirected," and "grim, dim canyons of our city streets," one can assume that the author is annoyed, offended, and disgruntled by modern architecture. Therefore, Choice *B,* aggrieved, is the most likely choice. None of the other answer choices accurately match the author's attitude.

Vocabulary

Etymology

By learning some of the etymologies (word origins) of words and their parts, readers can break new words down into components and analyze their combined meanings. For example, the root word *soph* is Greek for wise or knowledge. Knowing this informs the meanings of English words including *sophomore, sophisticated,* and *philosophy.* Those who also know that *phil* is Greek for love will realize that *philosophy* means the love of knowledge. They can then extend this knowledge of *phil* to understand *philanthropist* (one who loves people), *bibliophile* (book lover), *philharmonic* (loving harmony), *hydrophilic* (water-loving), and so on. In addition, *phob-* derives from the Greek *phobos,* meaning fear. This informs all words ending with it as meaning fear of various things: *acrophobia* (fear of heights), *arachnophobia* (fear of spiders), *claustrophobia* (fear of enclosed spaces), *ergophobia* (fear of work), and *hydrophobia* (fear of water), among others.

Some English word origins from other languages, like ancient Greek, are found in large numbers and varieties of English words. An advantage of the shared ancestry of these words is that once readers recognize the meanings of some Greek words or word roots, they can determine or at least get an idea of what many different English words mean. As an example, the Greek word *métron* means to measure, a measure, or something used to measure; the English word meter derives from it. Knowing this informs many other English words, including *altimeter, barometer, diameter, hexameter, isometric,* and *metric.* While readers must know the meanings of the other parts of these words to decipher their meaning fully, they already have an idea that they are all related in some way to measures or measuring.

While all English words ultimately derive from a proto-language known as Indo-European, many of them historically came into the developing English vocabulary later, from sources like the ancient Greeks' language, the Latin used throughout Europe and much of the Middle East during the reign of the Roman Empire, and the Anglo-Saxon languages used by England's early tribes. In addition to classic revivals and native foundations, by the Renaissance era other influences included French, German, Italian, and Spanish. Today we can often discern English word meanings by knowing common roots and affixes, particularly from Greek and Latin.

The following is a list of common prefixes and their meanings:

Prefix	Definition	Examples
a-	without	atheist, agnostic
ad-	to, toward	advance
ante-	before	antecedent, antedate
anti-	opposing	antipathy, antidote
auto-	self	autonomy, autobiography
bene-	well, good	benefit, benefactor
bi-	two	bisect, biennial
bio-	life	biology, biosphere
chron-	time	chronometer, synchronize
circum-	around	circumspect, circumference
com-	with, together	commotion, complicate
contra-	against, opposing	contradict, contravene

Prefix	Definition	Examples
cred-	belief, trust	credible, credit
de-	from	depart
dem-	people	demographics, democracy
dis-	away, off, down, not	dissent, disappear
equi-	equal, equally	equivalent
ex-	former, out of	extract
for-	away, off, from	forget, forswear
fore-	before, previous	foretell, forefathers
homo-	same, equal	homogenized
hyper-	excessive, over	hypercritical, hypertension
in-	in, into	intrude, invade
inter-	among, between	intercede, interrupt
mal-	bad, poorly, not	malfunction
micr-	small	microbe, microscope
mis-	bad, poorly, not	misspell, misfire
mono-	one, single	monogamy, monologue
mor-	die, death	mortality, mortuary
neo-	new	neolithic, neoconservative
non-	not	nonentity, nonsense
omni-	all, everywhere	omniscient
over-	above	overbearing
pan-	all, entire	panorama, pandemonium
para-	beside, beyond	parallel, paradox
phil-	love, affection	philosophy, philanthropic
poly-	many	polymorphous, polygamous
pre-	before, previous	prevent, preclude
prim-	first, early	primitive, primary
pro-	forward, in place of	propel, pronoun
re-	back, backward, again	revoke, recur
sub-	under, beneath	subjugate, substitute
super-	above, extra	supersede, supernumerary
trans-	across, beyond, over	transact, transport
ultra-	beyond, excessively	ultramodern, ultrasonic, ultraviolet
un-	not, reverse of	unhappy, unlock
vis-	to see	visage, visible

The following is a list of common suffixes and their meanings:

Suffix	Definition	Examples
-able	likely, able to	capable, tolerable
-ance	act, condition	acceptance, vigilance
-ard	one that does excessively	drunkard, wizard
-ation	action, state	occupation, starvation
-cy	state, condition	accuracy, captaincy
-er	one who does	teacher
-esce	become, grow, continue	convalesce, acquiesce
-esque	in the style of, like	picturesque, grotesque
-ess	feminine	waitress, lioness
-ful	full of, marked by	thankful, zestful
-ible	able, fit	edible, possible, divisible
-ion	action, result, state	union, fusion
-ish	suggesting, like	churlish, childish
-ism	act, manner, doctrine	barbarism, socialism
-ist	doer, believer	monopolist, socialist
-ition	action, result, state,	sedition, expedition
-ity	quality, condition	acidity, civility
-ize	cause to be, treat with	sterilize, mechanize, criticize
-less	lacking, without	hopeless, countless
-like	like, similar	childlike, dreamlike
-ly	like, of the nature of	friendly, positively
-ment	means, result, action	refreshment, disappointment
-ness	quality, state	greatness, tallness
-or	doer, office, action	juror, elevator, honor
-ous	marked by, given to	religious, riotous
-some	apt to, showing	tiresome, lonesome
-th	act, state, quality	warmth, width
-ty	quality, state	enmity, activity

Glossary of Important Terms

Abrasive: Someone who displays no concern over the feeling of others; irritating or harsh in manner. *Example:* The nurse found the patient in the waiting room to be rather abrasive.

Abstain: To refrain from doing something; to hold back. *Example:* They abstained from doing the surgery because the patient was displaying extreme anxiety.

Accountable: Responsible for. *Example:* The nurse was held accountable for forgetting to ask the patient for a full list of all current medications.

Acute: Of a serious or severe degree. *Example:* The patient experiencing acute pain was given specific instructions to follow on her medication.

Adhere: To comply with, follow, or stick together. *Example:* To adhere to the hospital's standards, the patients are permitted to enter the lounge only if they wear the proper equipment to prevent infection.

Adverse: In a negative or opposite way. *Example:* The patient's adverse reaction to the medication caused the doctor to prescribe an alternate medication.

Aegis: The protection of a certain organization or person. *Example:* Under the aegis of the medical board, nurses obtain certain rights in relation to their patients and themselves.

Ambivalent: Of a doubtful disposition. *Example:* The patient was ambivalent toward the idea of surgery the very next day.

Apply: To put on, to spread. *Example:* The doctor applied antibacterial ointment to the wound before covering it.

Assent: To approve or agree to something. *Example:* He wanted the child's assent before administering the shot.

Audible: Ability to be heard. *Example:* The girl's barely audible voice told us where the source of the pain was coming from.

Bacteria: A one-celled living organism; some are essential to forms of life, and some cause disease or death. *Example:* In order to kill the bacteria, doctors and nurses have a very specific way of washing their hands.

Bilateral: Affecting two sides of something. *Example:* The patient entered with bilateral ankle fractures.

Cardiac: Relating to the heart. *Example:* Sometimes preceding cardiac arrest, there will be weakness and heart palpitations, but sometimes sudden cardiac arrest will occur with no warning.

Cavity: An empty space or hole within the human body. *Example:* The nasal cavity has four different functions, one of which is to trap and remove pathogens from the air.

Cease: To cause to stop. *Example:* They had to cease administering the IV due to suspected clot formation.

Chronology: Arranging events according to the date. *Example:* Due to trauma that occurred, the chronology of events was difficult for the patient to remember.

Compensatory: To offset or make up for something. *Example:* The compensatory reaction to the patient's drop in blood pressure was the increase in his heart rate.

Concave: Shape that curves inward. *Example:* The concave appearance of the patient's chest suggested that the patient had *pectus excavatum*.

Concise: To be brief in one's information. *Example:* Notes written in order to display a patient's symptoms must be concise.

Consistency: How a liquid holds together; its thickness. *Example:* The consistency of the patient's mucous indicated there were flu-like symptoms present.

Constrict: When something comes together and is made smaller. *Example:* The patient's constricted throat indicated she was experiencing some kind of allergic reaction.

Contingent: Dependent upon something. *Example:* A healthy body is contingent upon eating well and exercising.

Contraindication: When a medical procedure is inadvisable because of a condition. *Example:* The surgery was contraindicated with the medication the patient was taking at the time.

Convulsive: Characterized by uncontrollable movements. *Example:* When the patient gained consciousness after their convulsive movements, they said everything was still fuzzy.

Cursory: Something done hastily. *Example:* The cursory inspection of the wound led to an erroneous diagnosis.

Defecate: To expel feces out of the body. *Example:* The patient was told to pay attention to how often they defecate within a day.

Deficit: A lack of something. *Example:* The personal trainer explained that the more intense the exercise, the more one would experience an oxygen deficit.

Depress: The motion downward. *Example:* To look inside the throat, place the tongue depressor on top of the tongue and hold down.

Depth: Distance from the surface down. *Example:* The doctor needed to find the depth of the wound in order to move forward in the treatment.

Deteriorating: To decline in function or health. *Example:* The patient's musculoskeletal system showed significant deterioration.

Device: A tool made for some specific purpose. *Example:* An insulin pump is a device used to administer insulin in the treatment of a person who is diabetic.

Diagnosis: An assessment to determine an illness or issue. *Example:* The doctor was sure that the diagnosis was kidney disease after she examined the patient a second time.

Dilate: To expand or become larger. *Example:* When he removed the light from her eyes, her pupils dilated back to normal.

Dilute: To make a liquid solution weaker, thinner, or less concentrated. *Example:* The patient was instructed to dilute hydrogen peroxide with water.

Discrete: Separate, apart from others. *Example:* The discrete scarring on the patient was cause for concern.

Distal: Away from the center of something, particularly the body. *Example:* The hand is distal to the shoulder.

Distended: Swollen or expanded due to pressure. *Example:* The patient underwent a series of tests for certain diseases that could cause a distended stomach.

Dysfunction: Functioning that is impaired or abnormal. *Example:* The paramedic concluded the woman was suffering from bowel dysfunction.

Empathy: The ability to understand and identify with the feelings of someone else. *Example:* One of the most important characteristics of therapists is the display of empathy towards their patients.

Equilibrium: A state of balance. *Example:* The patient's lack of equilibrium was said to be caused by Meniere's disease.

Etiology: Origin of a disease or condition. *Example:* The etiology of a patient's depression is said to be different in every case and includes possible traumatic events, health issues, and genetic vulnerability.

Exacerbate: To make worse. *Example:* The dentist said that sugary food and drink would exacerbate a cavity.

Expand: To widen or make bigger. *Example:* The expanding ring around the wound indicated that the area was getting infected.

Exposure: To be vulnerable to an outside source. *Example:* Exposure to certain bacteria while young can serve to protect children against diseases.

Extension: The act of lengthening a joint or limb. *Example:* The extension exercises the patient did for physical therapy helped them regain their flexibility.

External: On the outside of something. *Example:* The nurse gave the patient a topical medication that was for external use only.

Fatal: Leading to death. *Example:* The recently deceased was involved in a fatal accident that killed two other passengers.

Fatigue: A state of lethargy; to be tired. *Example:* The patient told the doctor he was experiencing extreme fatigue, headache, and chills.

Flexion: Act of bending a joint. *Example:* The flexion and extension exercises in physical therapy aided in the patient's ability to eventually walk.

Flushed: A red appearance in the skin, over the cheeks or neck. *Example:* He was flushed from heat exhaustion and dehydration.

Gastrointestinal: Having to do with the stomach or intestines. *Example:* Even though the patient's gastrointestinal tract looked normal, it was not functioning properly.

Hematologic: Relating to the blood. *Example:* Hemophilia is a hematologic disorder in which the blood is unable to clot normally.

Hydration: The act of absorbing water. *Example:* The dietician stressed the importance of hydration to aid in weight loss.

Hygiene: The practice of maintaining physical cleanliness. *Example:* Proper hygiene is an excellent way to prevent disease.

Impaired: To lack in function or have a disability. *Example:* The paramedics determined that the patient's eyesight was impaired due to the accident.

Impending: Forthcoming or about to happen. *Example:* The impending surgery was contingent on the patient's success in losing weight.

Impervious: Not allowing anything, such as liquids, to pass through. *Example:* Firefighters wear suits that are designed to be impervious to flames.

Imply: To suggest something. *Example:* The circular wound in the patient's chest and the amount of blood implied that the patient was a victim of a gunshot wound.

Incidence: An occurrence or rate of something. *Example:* The incidence of new strands of the flu every year is increasing at an alarming rate.

Infection: When the body becomes contaminated with pathogenic organisms. *Example:* The paramedic applied ointment to the infection.

Infer: To conclude something. *Example:* When the patient discussed her eating habits and body image, the dietician inferred that the patient was dealing with an eating disorder.

Inflamed: Swollen, and possibly red. *Example:* The nurse applied an ice pack to the patient's inflamed ankle.

Ingest: To take into the body food, drink, medicine, or some other substance by consuming or absorbing it. *Example:* The patient was told not to ingest any food or drink before surgery.

Initiate: To begin something. *Example:* The nurse initiated stricter protocols on the 5th floor.

Insidious: Something that happens gradually with harmful effects. *Example:* The disease was insidious, so the patient was almost too late in receiving treatment.

Intact: To be whole and in place. *Example:* Overall, the bone was intact and there would be no permanent damage.

Internal: On the inside of something. *Example:* Her internal organs were failing.

Invasive: The act of intrusion into a body part. *Example:* A catheter is an example of an invasive medical device.

Kinetic: Relating to movement. *Example:* Kinetic activities include dancing, running, and swimming.

Labile: Ability to change with frequency. *Example:* The patient was experiencing labile hypertension, which occurs when blood pressure fluctuates rapidly.

Laceration: A cut. *Example:* The patient had multiple lacerations from the train accident.

Latent: Something hidden or concealed. *Example:* Latent tuberculosis is where the TB infection in one's body remains inactive and displays no symptoms.

Lateral: Toward the side. *Example:* The patient had a lateral ankle sprain after the biking accident.

Lethargic: State of fatigue and sluggishness. *Example:* The dietician determined that the patient's lethargic state was due to an improper diet lacking in nutrients.

Manifestation: The appearance or sign of an ailment. *Example:* The doctor saw manifestations of celiac disease in the patient.

Musculoskeletal: Pertaining to both the musculature and skeletal system. *Example:* The musculoskeletal system is made up of ligaments, joints, bones, muscles, and cartilage, among other things.

Neurologic: Relating to the nervous system. *Example:* Many neurologic disorders can be treated with medications and rehabilitation.

Neurovascular: Relating to the nerves and blood vessels. *Example:* The patient was believed to have a neurovascular disorder.

Nutrient: A substance that is vital for growth and for the preservation of life. *Example:* The nutrients that come from fruits and vegetables are vital to health and wellbeing.

Occluded: To clog up or stop. *Example:* Blood clots are life-threatening because they have the potential to occlude oxygen flow in the body.

Ongoing: A state of continuance. *Example:* Managing ongoing conditions can be difficult, and a support group may be helpful to the affected patient.

Oral: Pertaining to the mouth. *Example:* The oral surgery was successful.

Otic: Pertaining to the ear. *Example:* The otic solution was effective in treating the patient's ear infection.

Parameter: The framework used to express or measure something. *Example:* The chart on the wall defines the parameter of high blood pressure.

Patent: To be open. *Example:* Since the wound was patent, the nurse had to take extra precaution in keeping it clean.

Pathogenic: A microorganism capable of causing disease. *Example:* A virus is a pathogenic organism that infects the living cells of a host.

Pathology: The behavior of a disease. *Example:* We had to study the pathology of Crohn's Disease in school.

Posterior: Referring to a place further back in position. *Example:* The bullet went through the front of the patient's right leg and exited through the posterior leg.

Potent: A strong effect. *Example:* The salts were potent enough to wake the patient from a fainting spell.

Potential: Possessing the ability to occur. *Example:* The doctor quickly noticed the patient's potential for a heart attack.

Precaution: A preventative measure. *Example:* The nurse took precaution before the surgery by washing her hands.

Precipitous: A swift or uncontrollable event. *Example:* The patient had experienced precipitous hearing loss.

Predispose: To be prone to a certain attitude or condition. *Example:* Some people are predisposed to depression due to family history.

Preexisting: A condition that exists prior to a certain time. *Example:* The patient's preexisting disease would be covered by medical insurance.

Primary: Relating to the first of something. *Example:* The paramedic's primary duty on the scene was to deliver CPR to the victim.

Priority: A thing of importance placed above everything else. *Example:* The nurse's first priority during the procedure was the patient's comfort.

Prognosis: The expected outcome of a disease. *Example:* The doctor spoke of a favorable prognosis for the patient's cancer.

Rationale: Relating to a logical basis of action. *Example:* It's important for the nurse to describe the rationale for taking the medication so that the patient will be more likely to follow the suggestion.

Recur: Something that happens repeatedly. *Example:* The patient described having trouble breathing as a recurring symptom.

Renal: Having to do with the kidneys. *Example:* Some patients suffering from renal disease will go through dialysis, a procedure that purifies the blood.

Respiration: Having to do with breathing. *Example:* The patient was in respiration distress.

Restrict: To limit the action of someone or something. *Example:* The patient was instructed to restrict his intake of salt for the next forty-eight hours.

Retain: To keep something. *Example:* In order to retain gum health, the dentist recommends using fluoride toothpaste.

Serene: Calm and tranquil. *Example:* The color of the hospital room and the flowers inside provided a serene atmosphere.

Status: The standing or condition of someone or something. *Example:* We could see the status of the patient's heart on the monitor.

Sublingual: Placed under the tongue. *Example:* The patient requested a sublingual vitamin because they had trouble swallowing pills.

Supplement: Something that is substituted by another thing. *Example:* The dietician suggested the patient supplement with Vitamin B12 since he was on a plant-based diet.

Suppress: The act of holding back or stopping. *Example:* The nurses were looking to suppress the patient's symptoms with antibiotics.

Symmetrical: Being the same on both sides. *Example:* The nurse found the two sides of the patient's face to still be symmetrical after the bandages were removed.

Symptom: A result of a disease or illness. *Example:* Her symptoms consisted of stiff, achy joints and fever.

Syndrome: Condition determined by associated symptoms. *Example:* After the patient displayed paralysis of eye muscles and loss of tendon reflexes, the doctor concluded she was suffering from Fisher's syndrome.

Therapeutic: Relating to the treatment of disease. *Example:* The amount needed to treat a disease is called a "therapeutic dose."

Toxic: Poisonous. *Example:* Toxic substances in the hospital must be disposed of in a certain way to avoid contamination.

Transdermal: Application of medicine through the skin. *Example:* The doctor gave the patient a transdermal patch to help with nicotine cravings.

Transmission: To transit something from one person to another. *Example:* The disease was high in potential transmission, so the staff took extra precautions with the patient.

Trauma: An injury. *Example:* The victim faced severe physical and emotional trauma from the accident.

Triage: The process of determining treatment order for patients based on the condition of the patient. *Example:* The hospital staff triaged the patients who arrived from the bus accident.

Ubiquitous: Being or seeming to be everywhere. *Example:* The patient described the pain as being ubiquitous.

Urinate: The act of releasing urine. *Example:* The patient was asked to urinate before the procedure.

Vascular: Pertaining to blood vessels. *Example:* The vascular system consists of vessels that carry blood throughout the body.

Verbal: Relating to spoken or unwritten words. *Example:* The verbal report included a concise plan for new treatment in the patient.

Virulent: Excessively harmful in its effects. *Example:* The patient was struggling to ward off the virulent disease.

Virus: An infective agent that multiplies in the cells of a living host. *Example:* The common cold is a virus that is characterized by coughing, sneezing, headache, runny nose, and fever.

Vital: Necessary. *Example:* It was vital that the paramedics did CPR when they first arrived on scene.

Volume: Amount of space of a liquid in a container. *Example:* The nurse measured the volume of the dose before giving it to the patient.

HESI Vocabulary Practice Questions

1. What is the meaning of the underlined word in the following sentence?

   The patient was <u>retained</u> for further observation.

   a. Made to leave
   b. Made to remain
   c. Led
   d. Accompanied

2. What is the best definition of the word *indication* in the following sentence?

   An elevated temperature is an <u>indication</u> of infection.

   a. Symptom
   b. Mistake
   c. Character
   d. Prognosis

3. Which of the following words is a synonym for the word *overt*?
   a. Obvious
   b. Concealed
   c. Central
   d. Annoying

4. What word meaning "writing down" fits best in the following sentence?

   The woman kept meticulous records by _____ each word correctly.

   a. Rewording
   b. Paraphrasing
   c. Shortening
   d. Transcribing

5. Choose the meaning of the underlined word in the following sentence:

   The board president <u>deterred</u> the committee from voting on the motion by dismissing it.

   a. Prevented
   b. Persuaded
   c. Assisted
   d. Contended with

6. Which word is an antonym for *dissuade*?
   a. Shave
   b. Adorn
   c. Appreciate
   d. Persuade

7. What is the best description for the word *integument*?
    a. Ligament
    b. Instrument
    c. Integrity
    d. Skin

8. Choose the meaning of the underlined word in the following sentence:

    The physician used a <u>hypodermic</u> needle for the injection.

    a. Above the skin
    b. Under the skin
    c. Disinfected
    d. Sterilized

9. What word means "to produce again"?
    a. Deduce
    b. Introduce
    c. Induce
    d. Reproduce

10. What word meaning "created" fits best in the following sentence?

    The writer _____ a document that detailed all of the happenings in the hospital.

    a. Discarded
    b. Adjourned
    c. Misaligned
    d. Composed

11. What is the best description for the word *hypothesis*?
    a. Conjecture
    b. Evidence
    c. Proof
    d. Research

12. Choose the meaning of the underlined word in the following sentence:

    The patient was having <u>labile</u> reactions to the medication.

    a. Changeable
    b. Accountable
    c. Dependable
    d. Lethal

13. Choose the word that is NOT a synonym for *contradict*.
    a. Negate
    b. Belie
    c. Repudiate
    d. Contractual

14. What word meaning "discern" fits best in the following sentence?

It was hard for the nurse to _____ whether the child was crying because she was afraid or sick.

a. Disengage
b. Distinguish
c. Disembowel
d. Dissociate

15. All EXCEPT which of the following words mean the same as *apprehensive*?
a. Foreboding
b. Timid
c. Trepid
d. Onerous

16. Choose the correct definition of the underlined word in the following sentence:

The man's initial symptoms were ultimately <u>unrelated</u> to his final diagnosis.

a. Pertinent
b. Admissible
c. Germaine
d. Irrelevant

17. Choose the meaning of the underlined word in the following sentence:

Several <u>salient</u> points emerged during the engaging presentation.

a. Scientific
b. Medical
c. Salivatory
d. Prominent

18. What is the best description for the word *nondescript*?
a. Ignorant
b. Exposed
c. Unassuming
d. Blatant

19. The man was removed from the room for making loud, derogatory comments about the attending physician. Describe the nature of the man's comments.
a. Enjoyable
b. Encouraging
c. Negative
d. Extensive

20. Choose the meaning of the underlined word in the following sentence:

Ultimately, the grandmother's choice to use unconventional medicine <u>superseded</u> the wishes of her children for more proven methods.

    a. Loathed
    b. Disdained
    c. Accredited
    d. Set aside

21. The opposite of the word *proximal* is _____.
    a. Dorsal
    b. Beneath
    c. Distal
    d. Ventral

22. *Assuage* is best defined as which of the following?
    a. Persuade
    b. Irritate
    c. Argue
    d. Soothe

23. Choose the meaning of the underlined word in the following sentence:

The surgical assistant prepared the necessary <u>vessels</u> for surgery.

    a. Receptacles
    b. Vehicles
    c. Veins
    d. Femurs

24. What word is most closely related to *malignant*?
    a. Virulent
    b. Benign
    c. Regular
    d. Banal

25. What is the definition of the underlined word in the following sentence?

The nurse's assistant applied a <u>splint</u> to the child's broken finger.

    a. A device used to apply medication
    b. A device used to stabilize an injury
    c. A device used to administer medication orally
    d. A device used to replace a missing limb

86

26. Choose the meaning of the underlined word in the following sentence:

The medical staff was given directives to administer <u>palliative</u> care to the dying patient during his final hours.

    a. Antispasmodic
    b. Urgent
    c. Analgesic
    d. Rheumatic

27. Choose the word or phrase that will make the following sentence grammatically correct:

The man's strange behavior caused his _____ ability to be called into question.

    a. Arrived
    b. Sustained
    c. Epistemic
    d. Attention

28. *Pallid* is best described as _____.
    a. Colorful
    b. Brilliant
    c. Pale
    d. Pink

29. Choose the meaning of the underlined word in the following sentence:

The custodian knew that the scheduled times for cleaning would be <u>invariable</u>.

    a. Consistent
    b. Intermittent
    c. Unpredictable
    d. Occasional

30. Choose the word that means "vomit."
    a. Populate
    b. Variance
    c. Evacuate
    d. Emesis

31. Indigestion is best described as _____.
    a. The tendency to walk without balance
    b. A constant tingling sensation in the extremities
    c. Discomfort in the digestive system
    d. The inability to control all bodily functions

32. *Shirk* is best defined as:
    a. Stoic
    b. Counsel
    c. Sharp
    d. Evade

33. Choose the meaning of the underlined word in the following sentence:

The <u>reverberation</u> of the glass as it broke on the ground lacerated the silence of the night.

    a. Reverence
    b. Resonance
    c. Berate
    d. Unison

34. Choose the meaning of the underlined word in the following sentence:

The reverberation of the sound of glass as it broke on the ground <u>lacerated</u> the silence of the night.

    a. Emasculated
    b. Beckoned
    c. Cut
    d. Slapped

35. Choose the word that means "to chew."
    a. Imbibe
    b. Peristalsis
    c. Masticate
    d. Cacophony

36. Choose the meaning of the underlined word in the following sentence:

The woman could not <u>deduce</u> the meaning of the entire conversation from the few words she overheard.

    a. Insult
    b. Avoid
    c. Decipher
    d. Measure

37. What word meaning "to tell again" best fits in the following sentence?

The woman felt the need to _____ the fact that she had asked to be discharged from the hospital several times.

    a. Chart
    b. Share
    c. Advance
    d. Reiterate

38. The word or phrase that is most closely related to the definition of the word *impotent* is _____.
    a. Stale
    b. Immovable
    c. Unable to perform
    d. Indicative

39. The definition of *exoskeleton* is _____.
    a. Internal organs
    b. An accumulation of cells
    c. External skeleton
    d. Skeletal fragments

40. *Alienation* is best described as _____.
    a. Adhesive
    b. Attachment
    c. Disapproval
    d. Isolation

41. Choose the meaning of the underlined word in the following sentence:

    The woman's <u>contractions</u> increased as her baby moved into the birth canal.

    a. Production
    b. Encapsulation
    c. The process in which muscles shorten
    d. Induction

42. Choose the meaning of the underlined word in the following sentence:

    The woman's contractions increased as her baby moved into the birth <u>canal.</u>

    a. Blockage
    b. Impact
    c. Passageway
    d. River

43. The definition of *relegate* is _____.
    a. Transition
    b. Classify
    c. Reassign to a lower position
    d. Envision

44. What is the best description for the word *castigate*?
    a. To remove the testicles
    b. Release
    c. Criticize
    d. Demand

45. Choose the meaning of the underlined word in the following sentence:

    The man had several <u>hematomas</u> after the minor car accident.

    a. Fractures
    b. Abrasions
    c. Bruises
    d. Tumors

46. The word most closely related to the definition of *adverse* is _____.
    a. Challenging
    b. Disgusting
    c. Affirming
    d. Unfavorable

47. The definition of the word *pharmaceutical* is _____.
    a. Of or relating to alcoholism
    b. Of or relating to medical terminology
    c. Of or relating to medication
    d. Of or relating to surgical procedures

48. *Cardiology* is described as the study of _____.
    a. The heart
    b. The lungs
    c. Blood
    d. The extremities

49. Choose the meaning of the underlined word in the following sentence:

    The teething baby's whimpering cries <u>elicited</u> hugs and sighs of sympathy from the mother.

    a. Prompted
    b. Denied
    c. Intimidated
    d. Evolved

50. Choose the meaning of the underlined word in the following sentence:

    Her <u>morose</u> countenance caused her to have difficulty making new friends.

    a. Radiant
    b. Expressive
    c. Sad
    d. Luminous

For each of the following questions, choose the one word whose meaning is MOST similar to the word printed in capital letters.

51. PROXIMITY
    a. Estimate
    b. Delicate
    c. Precarious
    d. Closeness

52. ADVOCATE
    a. Entice
    b. Brandish
    c. Decline
    d. Support

53. INCITE
   a. Calm
   b. Provoke
   c. Smell
   d. Repent

54. TACIT
   a. Unspoken
   b. Shortened
   c. Tenuous
   d. Regal

55. MOLLIFY
   a. Pacify
   b. Blend
   c. Negate
   d. Amass

Answer Explanations

1. B: Made to remain. Choice *A* is incorrect because *leaving* is the opposite of being *retained*. Choices *C* and *D* are also incorrect. The reader can infer from the example sentence that the patient wasn't being led and didn't require a companion for further observation.

2. A: Symptom. Choice *B* is incorrect because *mistake* does not make sense within the context of the sentence. Choice *C* is also incorrect because the word *character* refers to an individual's distinguishable qualities as a whole, not a single cause that led to an adverse result. Choice *D, prognosis,* might be an appealing choice because it does refer to diseases and medicine, but it refers to the expected outcome or course of a medical condition. A doctor may describe a favorable prognosis or a prognosis that is bleak, for example, depending on the condition. An elevated temperature, or fever, is not a prognosis but a symptom.

3. A: Obvious. The word overt can mean "obvious," "open," or "apparent." Choice *B* is incorrect; *concealed* is the opposite of the correct answer. Choices *C* and *D, central* and *annoying,* are incorrect.

4. D: Transcribing is most synonymous with writing down. Choices *A, B,* and *C* are all plausible because they are related to writing. However, Choice *D* is the correct answer because it pertains to recording what has been said instead of editing or revising it.

5. A: Prevented. Choices *B* and *C* are incorrect because the board president probably would not have persuaded or assisted the committee by dismissing a motion. Choice *D* is also incorrect. While the word *contend* has a negative connotation, a struggle or fight may not have resulted in a dismissed decision. *Deterred* means dissuaded or prevented.

6. D: Persuade. Choices *A, B,* and *C* are incorrect because *shave, appreciate,* and *adorn* are unrelated to the word *dissuade*. Choice *D* is correct because both words have the same root word, which means "to urge." The prefix *per-* means "thoroughly," and the prefix *dis-* means "not."

7. D: Skin. *Integument* is a skin or coating. The integumentary system in humans refers to our skin, hair, and nails. *Ligaments* are a type of connective tissue that attaches bone to bone. Choices *B* and *C* sound a bit like the word *integument,* but they do not have the same meaning.

8. B: Under the skin. Choices *C* and *D* are unrelated to *hypodermic*. Although all needles used in medical procedures should be sterilized to prevent the spread of bacteria, the term *hypodermic* is unrelated to the cleanliness of the needle. Choice *A* is a reasonable possibility because the root word *derm-* refers to skin, but it is also incorrect. The prefix *hypo-* refers to "under" or "beneath." Therefore, hypodermic means "under or below the skin."

9. D: Reproduce. Choices *A, B,* and *C* are incorrect because they are unrelated to production. Choice *D* is correct because the prefix *re-* means "to repeat," and the root word is *produce*.

10. D: Composed. Choices *A* and *B* are incorrect because both are related to ending something or throwing something away. Choice *C* does not make sense within the context of the sentence. Choice *D* is correct because *compose* means "to create or write."

11. A: Conjecture. Choices *B, C,* and *D* are related to research studies like the word *hypothesis,* but they are not synonymous with the word. Choice *A* is correct because *conjecture* is a formation of a theory or educated guess, just like a hypothesis. A scientist forms a hypothesis before conducting an experiment and designs the experiment to test the validity of the hypothesis.

12. A: *Labile* means likely to change, or unstable, so Choice *A* is correct. Choice *C* is a near antonym because something apt to change is not dependable. Choice *B* is incorrect; test takers who selected this choice may be confusing the word *labile* with *liable,* which does mean responsible or accountable. Choice *D* means deadly, so it is incorrect; though some adverse reactions to medications may be lethal, *labile* is not synonymous with *lethal.*

13. D: Contractual. Choices *A, B,* and *C* are all related to contradicting, or showing to be false, so these are incorrect because they are synonyms, not antonyms, of *contradict.* Choice *D* is correct because although it contains the *contra-* prefix, it refers to something related to a contract or under an agreement of sorts.

14. B: Distinguish. *Discern* means to distinguish or determine based on what can be seen. Choices *A* and *D* mean "to disconnect," so they are incorrect. Choice *C* means "to gut," as in removing the insides (bowels) of an animal.

15. D: Onerous. Choices *A, B,* and *C* are incorrect because they are all related to the word *apprehensive.* Choice *D* is correct because *onerous* means burdensome or troublesome. It usually is used to describe a task or obligation that may impose a hardship or burden, often which may be perceived to outweigh its benefits.

16. D: Irrelevant. Choices *A, B,* and *C* are all antonyms of *unrelated.* Choice *D* is correct because it describes the state of not pertaining or being related to a certain subject matter.

17. D: Prominent. Choices *A* and *B* are scientific terms that are unrelated to *salient.* Choice *C* looks similar to the word, but it is related to the gland that produces saliva, so it is incorrect. Choice *D* is correct because it is related to taking the forefront or eliciting increased engagement.

18. C: Unassuming. Choices *B* and *D, exposed* and *blatant,* both mean "to be recognizable," so these are incorrect. Choice *A* is incorrect because the word *ignorant* describes a lack of knowledge or awareness. Choice *C* is correct because it means "not apparent" or "not descriptive."

19. C: Negative. Choices *A* and *B, enjoyable* and *encouraging,* have a positive connotation and would not cause a person to be removed. Choice *D, extensive,* does not pertain to the situation. Therefore, Choice *C* is correct.

20. D: Set aside. Choices *A* and *B* both mean "to dislike," which is a plausible answer, since the children don't agree with their parent's decision. However, these are incorrect because they don't make sense within the sentence. Choice *C* is incorrect because it means "to give credit to something."

21. C: Distal. Choices *A* and *D, dorsal* and *ventral,* are both anatomical direction terms, meaning the top and bottom side of an animal, respectively. However, *proximal* means "close," and distal means "apart." In anatomy, a proximal structure is closer to the core and a distal one is further away on the extremity. For example, the ankle is distal to the knee.

22. D: *Assuage* most nearly means to soothe or comfort, as in to assuage one's fears. It can also mean to lessen or make less severe, or to relieve. For example, an ice pack on a swollen knee may assuage the pain.

23. A: Receptacles. Choices *C* and *D* are medically-related but incorrect because veins don't have to be prepped for surgery at all times. Additionally, the femur is a bone, so Choice *D* is incorrect. Choice *B*, *vehicles*, is unrelated in this context. Choice *A* is something that holds liquids or substances and fits best within the context of the sentence.

24. A: Virulent. *Malignant* means highly infectious or virulent. Tumors that tend to grow back or spread, particularly in the case of cancer, are often described as malignant, but infectious diseases can be as well. Choices *C* and *D*, *regular* and *banal*, mean "commonplace." Choice *B*, *benign*, means "harmless," so it is incorrect.

25. B: A device used to stabilize an injury. Choices *A* and *C* address administering medication but may not be what is necessary for a broken finger. Choice *D* refers to a prosthesis, which may be appealing in the case of a broken bone, but prostheses act as artificial limbs in cases where the patient has undergone an amputation or is missing a limb for other reasons. Choice *B* is the answer because the child's finger would need to be stabilized.

26. C: Palliative care focuses on the reduction of pain and making the patient comfortable. In this way, it is analgesic (pain-relieving) in its primary aim. Choice *A*, *antispasmodic*, refers to a drug used to combat muscle cramps. While some palliative care may involve such a medication, palliative care is mostly aimed at pain reduction, so this is not the best choice. Choice *B*, *urgent*, refers to immediate response care that may be more appropriate for a sudden onset illness. Choice *D*, *rheumatic*, doesn't make sense here because it refers to an affliction of the extremities or back (such as rheumatoid arthritis). Choice *C* is the correct answer because medical staff would focus on making the patient comfortable (free from pain) during their last hours.

27. C: Epistemic. Choices *A* and *D*, *arrived* and *attention*, don't make sense within the context of the sentence. Choice *B*, *sustained*, implies that his ability had been demonstrated continually, but the phrase *called into question* denotes a change. Choice *C* is the correct answer because *epistemic* refers to cognition. A change in actions may cause one's cognitive ability to be reevaluated.

28. C: Pale. Choices *A* and *B*, *colorful* and *brilliant*, are opposite of *pallid* because they denote a colorful hue. Choice *D* is not correct because *pink* is too specific. Choice *C* is correct because *pallid* means "pale" or "lacking color."

29. A: Consistent. Choices *B* and *D*, *intermittent* and *occasional*, are incorrect because they both refer to a gap in time frame. Choice *C*, *unpredictable*, is somewhat opposite the meaning of *invariable*. Choice *A* is the correct answer because the prefix *in-* means "not" in this instance, and the root word is *variable*. Therefore, *invariable* means "not varying" or "constant" or "consistent."

30. D: Emesis. Choices *A* and *B*, *populate* and *variance*, are not related to *vomit*. Choice *C*, *evacuate*, is also incorrect. Though the word *evacuate* means "to leave," the word *emesis* is a better fit here. The correct answer is *emesis*, which is the medical term used for *vomit*.

31. C: Discomfort in the digestive system. Choices *A* and *B* both address walking and extremities, which are not related to digestion. Choice *D* is incorrect because it is too inclusive when referring to *all bodily functions*. Choice *C* is correct because the prefix *in-* means "not" in this instance, and *digestion* refers to the process by which the body breaks down food. Therefore, indigestion would cause discomfort in the digestive system.

32. D: The word *shirk* means to evade and is often used in the context of shirking a responsibility, duty, or work.

33. B: Resonance. Choice *A* means a deep respect for someone, while Choice *C* means to harshly criticize, so these do not make sense. Choice *D* is highly unlikely, since glass probably wouldn't break in unison. Choice *B* is correct because breaking glass would cause a loud sound in a quiet room that might be prolonged or resonate for some time.

34. C: Cut. Choices *A* and *D* are incorrect because the sound could not be slapped or be deprived of its strength. Choice *B*, *beckoned*, means "to signal or summon," so this is also incorrect. Choice *C*, *cut*, is the correct answer, since the loud noise would figuratively "cut" the silence.

35. C: Masticate. Choice *A*, *imbibe*, means to drink (usually referring to alcohol). Choice *B*, *peristalsis*, refers to the wave-like contractions of smooth muscle along the digestive tract that move the bolus of food along. Choice *D*, *cacophony*, refers to an unpleasant sound or mix of discordant sounds but doesn't specifically refer to chewing. Therefore, Choice *C* is the correct answer because *masticate* means to chew.

36. C: Decipher. Choice *A*, *insult*, doesn't make sense within the context of the sentence. Choice *B*, *avoid*, is incorrect because the listener would not be trying to avoid the conversation while simultaneously trying to listen to what is being said. Choice *D*, *measure*, is not the best answer. Choice *C* is the correct answer because one deciphers or determines what was being said.

37. D: Reiterate. Choices *A* and *C*, *chart* and *advance*, don't make sense within the context of the sentence. Choice *B*, *share*, is a possibility, since the woman could share the information. However, sharing the fact several times makes Choice *D* the correct answer because *reiterate* means "to say or do something repeatedly."

38. C: Unable to perform. Choices *A* and *B*, *stale* and *immovable*, refer to something that doesn't move. Choice *D*, *indicative*, is not related. Impotent is often used in the context of sexual performance issues.

39. C: External skeleton. Choices *B* and *D* are incorrect because they are medical terminology that refer to parts of a whole. Furthermore, Choice *A*, internal organs, is not related to the skeleton. Choice *C* is correct because the prefix *exo-* refers to outside. Therefore, the exoskeleton is outside of the body.

40. D: Isolation. Choice *C*, *disapproval*, is not related. Choices *A* and *B*, *adhesive* and *attachment*, refer to the idea of being stuck together. Choice *D* is correct because *alienation* refers to being in isolation or set apart.

41. C: The process in which muscles shorten, causing pain. Choice *B*, *encapsulation*, means "the act of enclosing" and doesn't make sense within the context of the sentence. Choice *A*, *production*, is not specific enough. Though the word *induction* can be associated with labor and delivery, Choice *C* is the best fit because it refers to the contractions that cause the baby to move into the birthing canal.

42. C: Passageway. Choices *B* and *D*, *impact* and *river*, don't make sense within the sentence. Choice *A*, *blockage*, is incorrect because a blockage would keep the baby from moving. Choice *C* is correct because a *canal* is a passageway.

43. C: Reassign to a lower position. Choice *D, envision,* means "to picture mentally" and is therefore not related. Choices *A* and *B, transition* and *classify,* are too vague. Choice *C* is correct because *relegate* means "to move to a lower assignment or position."

44. C: *Castigate* means to correct harshly or criticize. Choice *A* is referring to *castration* not *castigate.* Choice *D* is incorrect; a *demand* is less specific than a correction. Therefore, Choice *C* is the correct answer because *castigate* means "to criticize or correct harshly."

45. C: Bruises. Choice *C* is correct because a hematoma is a bruise, or a collection of blood under the skin from broken blood vessels. The prefixes *hema-* and *hemato-* means blood. Choice *B, abrasions,* often involves blood because abrasions are scrapes on the skin. Although the suffix of *hematoma, -oma,* means a tumor or cancer (as in melanoma or carcinoma), a *hematoma* itself is not a tumor, but an abnormal subcutaneous buildup of blood.

46. D: Unfavorable. Choices *B* and *C, disgusting* and *affirming,* are not correct. Choice *A* is a possibility because it also has a negative connotation and is associated with struggle or difficulty. However, Choice *D* is the definition most closely related to the word *adverse.*

47. C: Of or relating to the sale or use of medication. Choice *A, of or relating to alcoholism,* is incorrect. Choices *B* and *D* are incorrect because, although they are associated with the medical field, they don't mention medicine. The prefix *pharma-* would denote that there is an association with medicine. For example, a pharmacy is where medications may be dispensed. Therefore, Choice *C* is correct.

48. A: The heart. Choices *B, C,* and *D* are incorrect because the prefix *cardio-* refers to the heart. Therefore, Choice *A* is the correct answer.

49. A: Prompted. Choice *D, evolved,* means "to develop gradually" and is therefore incorrect. Choices *B* and *C, denied* and *intimidated,* are incorrect because a mother would not likely ignore a crying child or be intimidated by the crying child. Choice *A* is correct because a crying child would prompt a response from the mother.

50. C: Sad. Choice *B, expressive,* is incorrect because someone with an expressive countenance would most likely not have difficulty with meeting other people initially. Choices *A* and *D, radiant* and *luminous,* are incorrect because the words mean the opposite of *morose,* which means "sad." Therefore, Choice *C* is the correct answer.

51. D: *Proximity* is defined as closeness, or the state or quality of being near in place, time, or relation.

52. D: To *advocate* means to *support* something or someone. Advocate here is presented as a verb; we see the verb *support* in the answer choices, which is the closest in meaning to *advocate.*

53. B: The word *incite* means to encourage or stir up disruptive behavior. A synonym for the word *incite* is *provoke,* which means to stimulate or stir up emotion in someone.

54. A: Something that is *tacit* is usually unspoken but implied. Tacit approval, for example, occurs when agreement or approval is understood without explicitly stating it.

55. A: *Mollify* means to soothe, pacify, or appease. It usually is used to refer to reducing the anger or softening the feelings or temper of another person, or otherwise calm them down. For example, a customer service associate may need to mollify an irate customer who is furious about the defect in their purchase.

Grammar

Eight Parts of Speech

Nouns

A **noun** identifies a person, animal, place, idea, or thing. The etymology of the word *noun* comes from the Latin *nomen*, which means "name." The two types of nouns are *common* or *proper* nouns. There are also collective nouns, abstract nouns, and concrete nouns.

The term **common noun** refers to nouns that are in a more general category of nouns, and to which **proper nouns** belong. For example, a common noun would be the word *teacher* or *professor*, while *Mrs. Smith* or *Professor Jones* would be considered proper nouns. Proper nouns will usually always be capitalized, so it's easier to tell common nouns from proper nouns. In the sentence below, the common nouns are in **bold**, and the proper nouns are in *italics*.

> *Keegan* wanted to go to a **university**, but she didn't want to go to just any **university**. *Duke University* was a **place** she always set her **eye** on, ever since she was a little **girl**. That was the **place** for her.

Notice how the common nouns like girl, place, and university, become proper nouns once they are specified and capitalized, like Duke University and Keegan.

Abstract nouns are nouns that designate a general concept or idea that is intangible. Below is a list of abstract nouns, expressing emotion, feeling, states, concepts, and events:

- Love
- Hate
- Bravery
- Compassion
- Integrity
- Beauty
- Justice
- Truth
- Thought
- Progress
- Friendship
- Relaxation
- Death

Concrete nouns are things people are capable of experiencing through the five senses. These are opposite of abstract nouns in that you can see, touch, hear, smell, or taste them. Here are some examples of concrete nouns:

- Table
- Student
- Teacher
- Pen
- University
- Storm

- Fruit
- Cat
- Mountain
- Park
- Gorilla
- Businessman
- Dentist

Collective nouns describe a group of individuals, animals, or things, and in American English, are paired with singular verbs, such as *The family is moving* or *The blue team wins the championship*. A list of collective nouns are as follows:

- Jury
- Team
- Family
- Audience
- Herd
- Band
- Swarm
- Army
- Colony
- Flock
- Group

Pronouns

Pronouns take the place of nouns in sentences. For example, in "John saw Mary, and he waved to her," "he" replaces "John," and "her" replaces "Mary." This reads much better than "John saw Mary, and John waved to Mary," which sounds repetitious. There are several different types of pronouns:

- Personal pronouns show the differences in person, gender, number, and case: he, she, they, it, we, him, her, us, them, I, you

- Demonstrative pronouns replace a noun phrase: this, these, that, those

- Interrogative pronouns are used to ask questions: which, who, whom, what, whose

- Indefinite pronouns do not refer to any one thing in particular: none, several, anything, something, anyone, everyone

- Possessive pronouns indicate possession: his, hers, theirs, mine, yours

- Reciprocal pronouns indicate that two or more people are acting in the same way towards the other: each other, one another

- Relative pronouns are used to connect phrases to a noun or pronoun: that, who whom, whose, which, whichever, whatsoever

- Reflexive pronouns are preceded by the adverb, adjective, or noun to which it refers: myself, yourself, himself, herself, oneself, itself, ourselves, themselves

Verbs

A **verb** is a word or phrase that expresses action, feeling, or state of being. Verbs explain what their subject is *doing*. Three different types of verbs used in a sentence are action verbs, linking verbs, and helping verbs.

Action verbs show a physical or mental action. Some examples of action verbs are *play, type, jump, write, examine, study, invent, develop,* and *taste*. The following example uses an action verb:

> Kat *imagines* that she is a mermaid in the ocean.

The verb *imagines* explains what Kat is doing: she is imagining being a mermaid.

Linking verbs connect the subject to the predicate without expressing an action. The following sentence shows an example of a linking verb:

> The mango *tastes* sweet.

The verb *tastes* is a linking verb. The mango doesn't *do* the tasting, but the word *taste* links the mango to its predicate, sweet. Most linking verbs can also be used as action verbs, such as *smell, taste, look, seem, grow,* and *sound*. Saying something *is* something else is also an example of a linking verb. For example, if we were to say, "Peaches is a dog," the verb *is* would be a linking verb in this sentence, since it links the subject to its predicate.

Helping verbs are verbs that help the main verb in a sentence. Examples of helping verbs are *be, am, is, was, have, has, do, did, can, could, may, might, should,* and *must,* among others. The following are examples of helping verbs:

> Jessica *is* planning a trip to Hawaii.
>
> Brenda *does* not like camping.
>
> Xavier *should* go to the dance tonight.

Notice that after each of these helping verbs is the main verb of the sentence: *planning, like,* and *go*. Helping verbs usually show an aspect of time.

Adjectives

Adjectives are descriptive words that modify nouns or pronouns. They may occur before or after the nouns or pronouns they modify in sentences. For example, in "This is a big house," *big* is an adjective modifying or describing the noun *house*. In "This house is big," the adjective is at the end of the sentence rather than preceding the noun it modifies.

A rule of punctuation that applies to adjectives is to separate a series of adjectives with commas. For example, "Their home was a large, rambling, old, white, two-story house." A comma should never separate the last adjective from the noun, though.

Adverbs

Whereas adjectives modify and describe nouns or pronouns, **adverbs** modify and describe adjectives, verbs, or other adverbs. Adverbs can be thought of as answers to questions in that they describe when, where, how, how often, how much, or to what extent.

Many (but not all) adjectives can be converted to adverbs by adding –*ly*. For example, in "She is a quick learner," *quick* is an adjective modifying *learner*. In "She learns quickly," *quickly* is an adverb modifying *learns*. One exception is *fast*. *Fast* is an adjective in "She is a fast learner." However, –*ly* is never added to the word *fast*; it retains the same form as an adverb in "She learns fast."

Prepositions

Words that show relationships between a noun or a pronoun and some other word are considered **prepositions**. Prepositional phrases begin with prepositions and end with nouns or pronouns, or the object of the preposition. For example: The cattle ran *over the hill*. The prepositional phrase is *over the hill*. The word *over* is the preposition, and the phrase *the hill* is the object of the preposition. Here is a list of prepositional words, although it is not comprehensive:

about	above	across	after	against	along
among	around	at	because of	before	behind
below	beneath	beside	between	despite	down
during	in front of	inside	into	near	off
onto	outside	over	past	through	toward
under	underneath	until	up	within	without

Prepositional phrases are useful in describing spatial temporal relations, like the following phrases including a box:

- Aside the box
- Under the box
- Inside the box
- Underneath the box
- Through the box
- Onto the box
- Over the box

Conjunctions

A **conjunction** is a word used to connect clauses or sentences, or the words used to connect words to other words. The words *and, but, or, nor, yet,* and *so* are conjunctions. Two types of conjunctions are called *coordinating conjunctions* and *subordinating conjunctions*.

Coordinating conjunctions join two or more items of equal linguistic importance. These conjunctions are *for, and, nor, but, or, yet,* and *so*, also called *FANBOYS* as an acronym. Here are each of the words used as coordinating conjunctions:

- They did not attend the reception that evening, for they were all sick from lunch.
- She bought a chocolate, vanilla, and raspberry cupcake.
- We do not eat pork, nor do we eat fish.
- I would bring her to the circus, but she is afraid of the clowns.

- She went to the grocery store, or she went to the park.
- Grandpa wanted to buy a house, yet he did not want to pay for it.
- We had a baby, so we bought a house on a lake.

Subordinating conjunctions are conjunctions that join an independent clause with a dependent clause. Sometimes they introduce adverbial clauses as well. The most common subordinating conjunctions in the English language are the following: *after, although, as, as far as, as if, as long as, as soon as, as though, because, before, even if, even though, every time, if, in order that, since, so, so that, than, though, unless, until, when, whenever, where, whereas, wherever,* and *while.* Here's an example of the subordinating conjunction, *unless.*

> Theresa was going to go kayaking on the river unless it started to rain.

Notice that "unless it started to rain" is the dependent clause, because it cannot stand by itself as a sentence. "Theresa was going to go kayaking on the river" is the independent clause. Here, *unless* acts as the subordinating conjunction, because the two clauses are not syntactically equal.

Interjections

An **interjection** is a word or expression that signifies a spontaneous emotion or reaction. Sometimes interjections stand by themselves and precede exclamation marks, such as "Wow!" "Yay!" or "Ouch!" Sometimes, interjections are used as hesitations markers, such as "er" or "um," and sometimes they are used as responses, such as "okay," "uh-huh," and "m-hmm."

Nine Important Terms to Understand

Clause

A **clause** is the smallest grammatical unit containing a subject and predicate. Two kinds of clauses are the independent clause and the dependent clause.

The **independent clause** can stand by itself as a complete sentence. It must contain a subject and a predicate at minimum, but it must not begin with a subordinating conjunction. The following two sentences are considered independent clauses:

> She swam.

> He ran to the edge of the sea and stuck his toe in.

Both of these are considered independent clauses because they express a complete thought. A **dependent clause** begins with a subordinating conjunction and is not considered a complete sentence, because it needs an independent clause to complete it. Let's add subordinating conjunctions to the sentences above and make dependent clauses:

> *Because* she swam.

> *Although* he ran to the edge of the sea and stuck his toe in.

These two sentences have become dependent on another idea due to the addition of subordinating conjunctions. Let's make these sentences complete by adding an independent clause:

Lilo was very healthy because she swam.

Although he ran to the edge of the sea and stuck his toe in, it was too cold to jump in.

Now these sentences consist of an independent clause and a dependent clause, which creates a complete sentence.

Direct Object

A **direct object** is directly affected by the action of the verb. In a sentence, the direct object usually answers the question *what* or *whom* and is the recipient of a transitive verb. The following is a simple sentence:

Ms. Shephard fed the cat.

Ms. Shephard is the subject, *fed* is the verb, and *the cat* is the direct object. *The cat* answers what Ms. Shephard fed. What did she feed? She fed the cat. Therefore, *the cat* is the direct object of the sentence.

Indirect Object

An **indirect object** refers to someone or something that is affected by the action of a transitive verb, such as the recipient of that action. To identify an indirect object, it is helpful to ask, "to whom was the thing received?" The following sentences contain examples of an indirect object in italics:

- She gave *him* the cat. (To whom did she give the cat? To him.)
- Mom gave *Bobby* a bath. (To whom did she give a bath? To Bobby.)
- Elijah made *Penelope* a cake. (To whom did he give a cake? To Penelope.)

In the above examples, recall the direct objects of each: *the cat, a bath*, and *a cake* are all direct objects of the sentence, while *him, Bobby,* and *Penelope* are the indirect objects of the sentence.

Phrase

A **phrase** is two or more words that stand together as a single unit. The difference between a phrase and a clause is that a clause contains the subject/verb pair, while a phrase does not. There are seven types of phrase examples listed below in italics:

- Noun phrase: made up of a noun and its modifiers. *"The astute, aged professor* started teaching again."

- Prepositional phrase: made up of a preposition and its object, and sometimes one or more adjectives. "I headed south *for the warm winters."*

- Participial phrase: begins with a past or present participial. The participial phrase serves as an adjective to the subject of the sentence. *"Having made up her mind to go to college,* Savannah took all the necessary classes for preparation."

- Gerund phrase: can be the subject of a sentence, the sentence's object, or the object of a preposition. Here is a gerund as the subject of a sentence: *"Swimming laps* was Harrison's favorite pastime."

- Infinitive phrase: phrase that begins with an infinitive ("to" + a verb). "My family loves *to vacation at the beach*."

- Appositive phrase: restates or describes a noun. "Dr. Masie, *the department chair in Chemistry*, is teaching the class."

- Absolute phrase: contains a subject but no acting verb. *"Her hands in the air*, she stared from the roller coaster into the dark tunnel."

Predicate

In a sentence, the **predicate** contains a verb and all the words that modify the verb. It is the part of the sentence that tells what is done by or done to the subject of the sentence. There are two examples of a predicate below:

The lady from the bakery *cooked the meal for us tonight*.

Destiny *wanted to be a surfer*.

A sentence, as a whole, is made up of a subject and a predicate. The predicate will always contain a verb, then any direct objects, indirect objects, or other phrases that come behind that verb.

Predicate Adjective

Predicate adjectives follow a linking verb and modify the subject of that linking verb. For example, when saying "the lamp is blue," *blue* is the predicate adjective of the sentence because it is an adjective that follows the linking verb *is* and modifies the subject *lamp*. In saying "thunderstorms have become scary," the word *scary* is the predicate adjective, because it modifies the subject *thunderstorms* and follows the linking verbs *have become*.

Predicate Nominative

A **predicate nominative** is the part of a sentence that completes the linking verb and renames the subject. For example, in the sentence "My favorite show is Game of Thrones," *Game of Thrones* is the predicate nominative because it renames "my favorite show" after the linking verb. Another example is saying "The places I have lived have been California, Texas, and Maine." *California, Texas,* and *Maine* are the predicate nominatives because they rename "the places I have lived" after the linking verb *have been*.

Sentence

By Purpose

Depending on the purpose of the sentence, one of four types will be used: declarative, imperative, interrogative, or exclamatory.

Declarative sentences are considered the most common of sentence types. Sentences like "I'm drinking coffee this morning," or "Kristin went to Europe this past summer" are declarative sentences.

Imperative sentences are sentences that make a command. Imperative sentences tell someone to do something, such as "Go to school!" or "Take out the trash."

Interrogative sentences ask questions or request information, such as "What does the first word of that sentence say?" or "Do you think I should try out for the dance team?"

Exclamatory sentences are statements that are more emotional, assertive, or energetic, and are usually marked by exclamation marks, such as "We won the championship!" or "I can't wait to go to Thailand!"

By Structure

When deconstructing sentences grammatically, there are four types of sentence structures: simple, compound, complex, and compound-complex.

Simple sentences contain a subject and a verb, and may contain additional phrases, indirect objects, or direct objects behind the sentence or verb. A simple sentence contains one independent clause only. Simple sentences can be as simple as saying, "Joanie laughed," or they can contain a compound subject, such as "Joanie and Marisa laughed." Simple sentences can also contain prepositional phrases and compound verbs, such as "Joanie and Marisa laughed at the movie and ate chocolate covered pretzels." Here we have a compound subject "Joanie and Marisa" and a compound verb "laughed and ate," yet we still have a single independent clause.

Compound sentences join two independent clauses together by a conjunction (for, and, nor, but, or, so). An example would be, "Zoe wanted to go to the zoo, but it was closed on Sundays." Here, we have two sentences that can stand on their own: "Zoe wanted to go to the zoo." "It was closed on Sundays." We could turn the simple sentence above into a compound sentence: "Joanie and Marisa laughed at the movie, and they ate chocolate covered pretzels." Adding "they" to the second part of the sentence creates two independent clauses. In a compound sentence, the FANBOYS are always separated by commas.

Complex sentences contain one independent clause and one dependent clause. As stated above, dependent clauses are similar to independent clauses; however, they lack some kind of unit that allows them to be a complete sentence. Dependent clauses may look like the following:

- When it started to rain
- After she bought the furniture for her new house
- Until the neighborhood street has a bike lane

In order to make these into complex sentences, we must attach independent clauses to each, either before or after the dependent clause. Here are some examples of a complex sentence:

- When it started to rain, Mazey shut all the windows except the one in the living room.
- Carolynn was ecstatic after she bought the furniture for her new house.
- Until the neighborhood street has a bike lane, I would prefer to take Charlie to the park.

Notice that the independent clauses are able to stand on their own, while the dependent clauses depend on the independent clause to complete the thought.

Compound-complex sentences occur when a complex sentence is merged with a compound sentence. These sentences have two independent clauses and one dependent clause. In the following examples, the dependent clauses are in bold, while the independent clauses are in italics:

- **When it started to rain**, *Mazey shut all the windows except the one in the living room*, and *her brother got out a board game to play.*

- *Carolynn was ecstatic* **after she bought the furniture for her new house**, but *she returned two pieces a day later.*

- **Until the neighborhood street has a bike lane**, *I would prefer to take Charlie to the park to ride his new bike*, for *this road is too busy to ride on.*

For fluent composition, writers must use a variety of sentence types and structures, and also ensure that they smoothly flow together when they are read. One way writers can increase fluency is by varying the beginnings of sentences. Writers do this by starting most of their sentences with different words and phrases rather than monotonously repeating the same ones across multiple sentences. Another way writers can increase fluency is by varying the lengths of sentences. Since run-on sentences are incorrect, writers make sentences longer by also converting them from simple to compound, complex, and compound-complex sentences. The coordination and subordination involved in these also give the text more variation and interest, hence more fluency. Here are a few more ways writers can increase fluency:

- Varying the transitional language and conjunctions used makes sentences more fluent.
- Writing sentences with a variety of rhythms by using prepositional phrases.
- Varying sentence structure adds fluency.

Subject

The **subject of the sentence** is the word or phrase that is being discussed or described relating to the verb. The ***complete subject*** is a subject with all its parts, like the following: *The stormy weather* ruined their vacation. A **simple subject** is the subject with all the modifiers removed. In the previous example the simple subject would be *weather.* There are various forms of subjects listed below:

- Noun (phrase) or pronoun: *The tiny bird* sang all morning long.
- A to-infinitive clause: *To hike the Appalachian Trail* was her lifelong goal.
- A gerund: *Running* was his new favorite sport.
- A that-clause: *That she was old* did not stop her from living her life.
- A direct quotation: *"Here comes the sun"* is a quote from a Beatle's song.
- A free relative clause: *Whatever she said* is none of my business.
- Implied subject: *(You)* Shut the door!

Ten Common Grammatical Mistakes

Subject-Verb Agreement

Lack of **subject-verb agreement** is a very common grammatical error. One of the most common instances is when people use a series of nouns as a compound subject with a singular instead of a plural verb. Here is an example:

> Identifying the best books, locating the sellers with the lowest prices, and paying for them *is* difficult

instead of saying "*are* difficult." Additionally, when a sentence subject is compound, the verb is plural:

> He and his cousins *were* at the reunion.

However, if the conjunction connecting two or more singular nouns or pronouns is "or" or "nor," the verb must be singular to agree:

> That pen or another one like it is in the desk drawer.

If a **compound subject** includes both a singular noun and a plural one, and they are connected by "or" or "nor," the verb must agree with the subject closest to the verb: "Sally or her sisters go jogging daily"; but "Her sisters or Sally goes jogging daily."

Simply put, **singular subjects** require singular verbs and plural subjects require plural verbs. A common source of agreement errors is not identifying the sentence subject correctly. For example, people often write sentences incorrectly like, "The group of students *were* complaining about the test." The subject is not the plural "students" but the singular "group." Therefore, the correct sentence should read, "The group of students *was* complaining about the test." The converse also applies, for example, in this incorrect sentence: "The facts in that complicated court case *is* open to question." The subject of the sentence is not the singular "case" but the plural "facts." Hence the sentence would correctly be written: "The facts in that complicated court case *are* open to question." New writers should not be misled by the distance between the subject and verb, especially when another noun with a different number intervenes as in these examples. The verb must agree with the subject, not the noun closest to it.

Comma in a Compound Sentence

To review, a compound sentence contains two independent clauses, like the following:

> Stacie was late to the meeting, and she forgot her briefcase.

The two clauses above can stand on their own as independent clauses if separated. This makes the above sentence a compound sentence.

Comma placement is important in compound sentences; commas always go before the conjunction. In the case above, the conjunction is *and*. Notice how there's a comma before *and*.

If we take out the "she" in the above sentence, the sentence is no longer a compound sentence. It becomes a simple sentence with a compound predicate:

> Stacie was late to the meeting and forgot her briefcase.

The compound predicate is "was late" and "forgot." Notice how, since the sentence is no longer a compound sentence, we no longer need the comma before *and*. If we add the *she* back in and join two independent clauses, we would have to reinsert the comma before the second independent clause.

Run-On Sentence

A **run-on sentence** combines two or more complete sentences without punctuating them correctly or separating them. For example, the following is a run-on sentence caused by a lack of punctuation:

> There is a malfunction in the computer system however there is nobody available right now who knows how to troubleshoot it.

One correction is, "There is a malfunction in the computer system; however, there is nobody available right now who knows how to troubleshoot it." Another is, "There is a malfunction in the computer system. However, there is nobody available right now who knows how to troubleshoot it."

An example of a comma splice is the following:

> Jim decided not to take the bus, he walked home.

Replacing the comma with a period or a semicolon corrects this. Commas that try and separate two independent clauses without a contraction are considered comma splices.

Pronoun Case

There are three **pronoun cases**: subjective case, objective case, and possessive case. Pronouns as subjects are pronouns that replace the subject of the sentence, such as *I, you, he, she, it, we, they* and *who*. Pronouns as objects replace the object of the sentence, such as *me, you, him, her, it, us, them,* and *whom*. Pronouns that show possession are *mine, yours, hers, its, ours, theirs,* and *whose*. The following are examples of different pronoun cases:

- Subject pronoun: *She* ate the cake for her birthday. *I* saw the movie.
- Object pronoun: You gave *me* the card last weekend. She gave the picture to *him*.
- Possessive pronoun: That bracelet you found yesterday is *mine*. *His* name was Casey.

Comma in a Series

Commas separate words or phrases in a series of three or more. The Oxford comma is the last comma in a series. Many people omit this last comma, but many times it causes confusion. Here is an example:

> I love my sisters, the Queen of England and Madonna.

This example without the comma implies that the "Queen of England and Madonna" are the speaker's sisters. However, if the speaker was trying to say that they love their sisters, the Queen of England, as well as Madonna, there should be a comma after "Queen of England" to signify this.

Commas also separate two coordinate adjectives ("big, heavy dog") but not cumulative ones, which should be arranged in a particular order for them to make sense ("beautiful ancient ruins").

Here are some brief rules for commas:

- Commas follow introductory words like *however, furthermore, well, why,* and *actually,* among others.

- Commas go between city and state: Houston, Texas.

- If using a comma between a surname and Jr. or Sr. or a degree like M.D., also follow the whole name with a comma: "Martin Luther King, Jr., wrote that . . ."

- A comma follows a dependent clause at the beginning of a sentence: "Although she was very small, . . ."

- Nonessential modifying words/phrases/clauses are enclosed by commas: "Wendy, who is Peter's sister, closed the window."

- Commas introduce or interrupt direct quotations: "She said, 'I hate him.' 'Why,' I asked, 'do you hate him?'"

Unclear or Vague Pronoun Reference

Pronouns within a sentence must refer specifically to one noun, known as the *antecedent*. Sometimes, if there are multiple nouns within a sentence, it may be difficult to ascertain which noun belongs to the pronoun. It's important that the pronouns always clearly reference the nouns in the sentence so as not to confuse the reader. Here's an example of an unclear pronoun reference:

> After Catherine cut Libby's hair, David bought her some lunch.

The pronoun in the examples above is *her*. The pronoun could either be referring to *Catherine* or *Libby*. Here are some ways to write the above sentence with a clear pronoun reference:

> After Catherine cut Libby's hair, David bought Libby some lunch.

> David bought Libby some lunch after Catherine cut Libby's hair.

But many times, the pronoun will clearly refer to its antecedent, like the following:

> After David cut Catherine's hair, he bought her some lunch.

Sentence Fragments

Sentence fragments are caused by absent subjects, absent verbs, or dangling/uncompleted dependent clauses. Every sentence must have a subject and a verb to be complete. An example of a fragment is the following:

> Raining all night long.

In the above example, there is no subject present. "It was raining all night long" is one correction. Another example of a sentence fragment is the second part in the following statement:

> Many scientists think in unusual ways. Einstein, for instance.

The second phrase is a fragment because it has no verb. One correction is "Many scientists, like Einstein, think in unusual ways." Finally, look for "cliffhanger" words like *if, when, because,* or *although* that introduce dependent clauses, which cannot stand alone without an independent clause. For example, to correct the sentence fragment "If you get home early," add an independent clause: "If you get home early, we can go dancing."

Misplaced Modifier

A **misplaced modifier** is a word, clause, or phrase that refers to an unintended word. Most modifiers can be edited to where they clearly modify the intended word instead of remaining ambiguous. Examples of misplaced modifiers are misplaced adjectives, adverb placement, misplaced phrases, and misplaced clauses. In the examples below, the modifiers are in bold, and the words they modify are in italics.

Misplaced adjectives are adjectives that are intended to modify nouns, but are actually separated from them. Misplaced adjectives can be easily corrected by positioning the adjective beside the noun it modifies. The following is an example followed by a correction:

Incorrect: Grandma ate a **warm** bowl of *soup* for dinner.

Correct: Grandma ate a bowl of **warm** *soup* for dinner.

If spoken in colloquial language, the first sentence would sound pretty accurate. We use misplaced adjectives all the time and they don't *seem* incorrect. However, in the above example, the soup is the thing that is warm, first and foremost, so the adjective should reflect that.

Adverb placement within a sentence can also turn into a misplaced modifier. Depending on where certain adverbs are placed, the meaning of the whole sentence can change. Here are adverb placements that can result in two different meanings:

Meaning 1: She **quickly** *vacuumed* the rug she had bought.

Meaning 2: She vacuumed the rug she had *bought* **quickly**.

The placement of the adverb *quickly* determines the meaning of the sentence. In the first example, we are told that she vacuumed the rug quickly. In the second sentence, we are told that she bought the rug quickly. Test takers should be aware of where they place their adverbs so to avoid confusion.

Misplaced phrases are phrases within a sentence that should be rearranged to create clarity. The following is an example of a misplaced phrase with the corrected phrase underneath:

Incorrect: The man gave the *vacation house* to his daughter **with the orange trees**.

Correct: The man gave the *vacation house* **with the orange trees** to his daughter.

The correct sentence places the modifying phrase next to the noun it modifies. In the first sentence, the logic of the sentence tells us that the daughter had the orange trees; the second sentence is corrected to tell us that it's the house that has the orange trees, not the daughter.

Misplaced clauses occur when a clause is modifying an incorrect noun. Below is an example of a misplaced clause:

Incorrect: The restaurant prepared a *dish* for the man **that was cooked in steamed milk**.

Correct: The restaurant prepared a *dish* **that was cooked in steamed milk** for the man.

In the first sentence, the logic of the sentence tells us that there was a man who was cooked in steamed milk, and the restaurant prepared a dish for him! To correct this error, place the clause next to the noun it is supposed to modify. In the corrected version, we see that it's the *dish* that was cooked in steamed milk, not the man.

Prepositions at the End of a Sentence

The avoidance of ending sentences with a preposition is thought to be an archaic rule from rhetoricians in the 17th century, stemming from the Latin language. Contemporary usage of the English language tells us that there are many instances where prepositions are the appropriate choice at the end of a sentence. The Oxford Dictionary website tells us four specific instances that are used:

- Passive structures: The deli on 43rd street *was broken into.*
- Infinitive structures: Ever since Katy moved to Iowa, she has found no one *to hang out with.*
- Relative clauses: She adored the pets *that her sister took care of.*
- Questions beginning with *who, where, what*, etc.: What kind of school are you going to?

Five Suggestions for Success

Eliminating Clichés and Euphemisms

In order for writers to sound original and fresh, they should avoid using clichés. **Clichés** are once-clever phrases that have been overused to the point where they have become imitative and dull. The following is a list of clichés that are popular today:

- The grass is always greener on the other side.
- A bird in the hand is worth two in the bush.
- Actions speak louder than words.
- Don't judge a book by its cover.
- Ignorance is bliss.
- I always bend over backwards for you.
- It's always calm before the storm.
- Good things come to those who wait.

A **euphemism** is a phrase used in place of another phrase usually viewed as harsh, inappropriate, or embarrassing. Below if a list of euphemisms and their counterparts:

- *Passed away* instead of died
- *Let go* instead of fired
- *Break wind* instead of pass gas
- The birds and the bees instead of sex
- *Curvy* instead of overweight
- Correctional facility instead of prison
- *Under the weather* instead of fallen sick
- *Couch potato* instead of lazy

Eliminating Sexist Language, Profanity, and Insensitive Language

Most sexist language that exists in English today is very subtle and is often socially constructed rather than individually biased. In the past, the correct pronoun to use to represent all humans was the universal *he*; now we are encouraged to use *he or she* (or sometimes *they*), or *humankind* instead of *mankind*. The use of sexist language creates a divide in gender equality and has the power to perpetuate oppressive gender assumptions. If we continually use the pronoun *he* to refer to doctors, we are suggesting that women *are not* or *should not be* included in that profession. Changing our pronoun use to include *she* in addition to *he* creates an atmosphere of inclusiveness and recognition. Using titles without gender, when possible, also serves to eliminate sexist language. An example of this would be to use *nurse* instead of *male nurse*, or *flight attendant* instead of *stewardess*.

110

Profanity and insensitive language is a definite way to offend your audience and turn them off of your writing. Profanity includes curse words used in certain contexts. Insensitive language is usually language directed toward a race, disability, gender, sexual orientation, age, or religion that intentionally or unintentionally offends or harms that particular category of people. At times, with language undergoing such rapid changes in our technological age, it is difficult to know what terms are appropriate to use and when we've offended someone. A quick search will usually tell us appropriate language to use, or it might even be appropriate to ask for help when uncertain of a word or phrase. As writers, it's important for us to be sensitive to words or phrases that may hurt groups of people.

Properly Using Homonyms, Homophones, and Homographs

Homophones are words that sound the same in speech, but have different spellings and meanings. For example, *to, too,* and *two* all sound alike, but have three different spellings and meanings. Homophones with different spellings are also called **heterographs**. **Homographs** are words that are spelled identically, but have different meanings. If they also have different pronunciations, they are **heteronyms**. For instance, *tear* pronounced one way means a drop of liquid formed by the eye; pronounced another way, it means to rip. Homophones that are also homographs are **homonyms**. For example, *bark* can mean the outside of a tree or a dog's vocalization; both meanings have the same spelling. *Stalk* can mean a plant stem or to pursue and/or harass somebody; these are spelled and pronounced the same. *Rose* can mean a flower or the past tense of *rise*. Many non-linguists confuse things by using "homonym" to mean sets of words that are homophones but not homographs, and also those that are homographs but not homophones.

The word *row* can mean to use oars to propel a boat; a linear arrangement of objects or print; or an argument. It is pronounced the same with the first two meanings, but differently with the third. Because it is spelled identically regardless, all three meanings are homographs. However, the two meanings pronounced the same are homophones, whereas the one with the different pronunciation is a heteronym. By contrast, the word *read* means to peruse language, whereas the word *reed* refers to a marsh plant. Because these are pronounced the same way, they are homophones; because they are spelled differently, they are heterographs. Homonyms are both homophones and homographs—pronounced and spelled identically, but with different meanings. One distinction between homonyms is of those with separate, unrelated etymologies, called "true" homonyms, e.g. *skate* meaning a fish or *skate* meaning to glide over ice/water. Those with common origins are called polysemes or polysemous homonyms, e.g. the *mouth* of an animal/human or of a river.

Developing Well-Organized Paragraphs

A **paragraph** is a series of connected and related sentences addressing one topic. Writing good paragraphs benefits writers by helping them to stay on target while drafting and revising their work. It benefits readers by helping them to follow the writing more easily. Regardless of how brilliant their ideas may be, writers who do not present them in organized ways will fail to engage readers—and fail to accomplish their writing goals. A fundamental rule for paragraphing is to confine each paragraph to a single idea. When writers find themselves transitioning to a new idea, they should start a new paragraph. However, a paragraph can include several pieces of evidence supporting its single idea; and it can include several points if they are all related to the overall paragraph topic. When writers find each point becoming lengthy, they may choose instead to devote a separate paragraph to every point and elaborate upon each more fully.

An effective paragraph should have these elements:

- Unity: One major discussion point or focus should occupy the whole paragraph from beginning to end.

- Coherence: For readers to understand a paragraph, it must be coherent. Two components of coherence are logical and verbal bridges. In logical bridges, the writer may write consecutive sentences with parallel structure or carry an idea over across sentences. In verbal bridges, writers may repeat key words across sentences. Parallel structure in a sentence matches the forms of sentence components. Any sentence containing more than one description or phrase should keep them consistent in wording and form. Readers can easily follow writers' ideas when they are written in parallel structure, making it an important element of correct sentence construction. For example, this sentence lacks parallelism: "Our coach is a skilled manager, a clever strategist, and works hard." The first two phrases are parallel, but the third is not. Correction: "Our coach is a skilled manager, a clever strategist, and a hard worker." Now all three phrases match in form.

- A topic sentence: The paragraph should have a sentence that generally identifies the paragraph's thesis or main idea.

- Sufficient development: To develop a paragraph, writers can use the following techniques after stating their topic sentence:

- Define terms
- Cite data
- Use illustrations, anecdotes, and examples
- Evaluate causes and effects
- Analyze the topic
- Explain the topic using chronological order

A **topic sentence** identifies the main idea of the paragraph. Some are explicit, some implicit. The topic sentence can appear anywhere in the paragraph. However, many experts advise beginning writers to place each paragraph topic sentence at or near the beginning of its paragraph to ensure that their readers understand what the topic of each paragraph is. Even without having written an explicit topic sentence, the writer should still be able to summarize readily what subject matter each paragraph addresses. The writer must then fully develop the topic that is introduced or identified in the topic sentence. Depending on what the writer's purpose is, they may use different methods for developing each paragraph.

Two main steps in the process of organizing paragraphs and essays should both be completed after determining the writing's main point, while the writer is planning or outlining the work. The initial step is to give an order to the topics addressed in each paragraph. Writers must have logical reasons for putting one paragraph first, another second, etc. The second step is to sequence the sentences in each paragraph. As with the first step, writers must have logical reasons for the order of sentences. Sometimes the work's main point obviously indicates a specific order.

To be effective, a topic sentence should be concise so that readers get its point without losing the meaning among too many words. As an example, in *Only Yesterday: An Informal History of the 1920s* (1931), author Frederick Lewis Allen's topic sentence introduces his paragraph describing the 1929 stock market crash: "The Bull Market was dead." This example illustrates the criteria of conciseness and brevity. It is also a strong sentence, expressed clearly and unambiguously. The topic sentence also introduces the paragraph, alerting the reader's attention to the main idea of the paragraph and the subject matter that follows the topic sentence.

Experts often recommend opening a paragraph with the topic sentences to enable the reader to realize the main point of the paragraph immediately. Application letters for jobs and university admissions also benefit from opening with topic sentences. However, positioning the topic sentence at the end of a paragraph is more logical when the paragraph identifies a number of specific details that accumulate evidence and then culminates with a generalization. While paragraphs with extremely obvious main ideas need no topic sentences, more often—and particularly for students learning to write—the topic sentence is the most important sentence in the paragraph. It not only communicates the main idea quickly to readers; it also helps writers produce and control information.

Using Conventions of Standard English Punctuation

Writing that adheres to the conventions of standard English punctuation is clear, coherent, and understandable to the reader. Strong writers appreciate that proper punctuation not only presents a more polished and professional piece, but also helps convey the intending meaning of the language used. In addition to the explanation about proper comma use and other punctuation marks previously discussed, the following information should help inform test takers about the grammatical conventions surrounding punctuation:

Ellipses

Ellipses (. . .) signal omitted text when quoting. Some writers also use them to show a thought trailing off, but this should not be overused outside of dialogue. An example of an ellipsis would be if someone is quoting a phrase out of a professional source but wants to omit part of the phrase that isn't needed: "Dr. Skim's analysis of pollen inside the body is clearly a myth . . . that speaks to the environmental guilt of our society."

Semicolons

Semicolons are used to connect two independent clauses, but should never be used in the place of a comma. They can replace periods between two closely connected sentences: "Call back tomorrow; it can wait until then." When writing items in a series and one or more of them contains internal commas, separate them with semicolons, like the following:

People came from Springfield, Illinois; Alamo, Tennessee; Moscow, Idaho; and other locations.

Hyphens

Here are some rules concerning hyphens:

- Compound adjectives like state-of-the-art or off-campus are hyphenated.
- Original compound verbs and nouns are often hyphenated, like "throne-sat," "video-gamed," "no-meater."
- Adjectives ending in –ly are often hyphenated, like "family-owned" or "friendly-looking."
- "Five years old" is not hyphenated, but singular ages like "five-year-old" are.
- Hyphens can clarify. For example, in "stolen vehicle report," "stolen-vehicle report" clarifies that "stolen" modifies "vehicle," not "report."
- Compound numbers twenty-one through ninety-nine are spelled with hyphens.
- Prefixes before proper nouns/adjectives are hyphenated, like "mid-September" and "trans-Pacific."

Parentheses

Parentheses enclose information such as an aside or more clarifying information: "She ultimately replied (after deliberating for an hour) that she was undecided." They are also used to insert short, in-text definitions or acronyms: "His FBS (fasting blood sugar) was higher than normal." When parenthetical information ends the sentence, the period follows the parentheses: "We received new funds ($25,000)." Only put periods within parentheses if the whole sentence is inside them: "Look at this. (You'll be astonished.)" However, this can also be acceptable as a clause: "Look at this (you'll be astonished)." Although parentheses appear to be part of the sentence subject, they are not, and do not change subject-verb agreement: "Will (and his dog) was there."

Quotation Marks

Quotation marks are typically used when someone is quoting a direct word or phrase someone else wrote or said. Additionally, quotation marks should be used for the titles of poems, short stories, songs, articles, chapters, and other shorter works. When quotations include punctuation, periods and commas should *always* be placed inside of the quotation marks.

When a quotation contains another quotation inside of it, the outer quotation should be enclosed in double quotation marks and the inner quotation should be enclosed in single quotation marks. For example: "Timmy was begging, 'Don't go! Don't leave!'" When using both double and single quotation marks, writers will find that many word-processing programs may automatically insert enough space between the single and double quotation marks to be visible for clearer reading. But if this is not the case, the writer should write/type them with enough space between to keep them from looking like three single quotation marks. Additionally, non-standard usages, terms used in an unusual fashion, and technical terms are often clarified by quotation marks. Here are some examples:

My "friend," Dr. Sims, has been micromanaging me again.

This way of extracting oil has been dubbed "fracking."

Apostrophes

One use of the **apostrophe** is followed by an *s* to indicate possession, like *Mrs. White's home* or *our neighbor's dog*. When using the *'s* after names or nouns that also end in the letter *s*, no single rule applies: some experts advise adding both the apostrophe and the *s*, like "the Jones's house," while others prefer using only the apostrophe and omitting the additional *s*, like "the Jones' house." The wisest expert advice is to pick one formula or the other and then apply it consistently. Newspapers and magazines often use *'s* after common nouns ending with *s*, but add only the apostrophe after proper nouns or names ending with *s*. One common error is to place the apostrophe before a name's final *s* instead of after it: "Ms. Hasting's book" is incorrect if the name is Ms. Hastings.

Plural nouns should not include apostrophes (e.g. "apostrophe's"). Exceptions are to clarify atypical plurals, like verbs used as nouns: "These are the do's and don'ts." Irregular plurals that do not end in *s* always take apostrophe-*s*, not *s*-apostrophe—a common error, as in "childrens' toys," which should be "children's toys." Compound nouns like mother-in-law, when they are singular and possessive, are followed by apostrophe-*s*, like "your mother-in-law's coat." When a compound noun is plural and possessive, the plural is formed before the apostrophe-*s*, like "your sisters-in-laws' coats." When two people named possess the same thing, use apostrophe-*s* after the second name only, like "Dennis and Pam's house."

Fifteen Troublesome Word Pairs

Affect versus Effect

The word *affect* is a verb, and it means to have an effect on something or to influence something. *Affect* is sometimes used as a noun, and in this way, it means an emotional response or disposition. The word *effect* is mostly used as a noun, and it refers to the impact or result of something. However, *effect* can also be used as a verb, meaning to cause something to come into being. Replacing the verb *effect* with *bring about* is useful in determining which word to use. Here are four examples of these words used correctly:

- Affect as verb: Her bravery the night before *affected* the way her peers treated her.
- Affect as noun: He had a moody *affect* during his everyday routines.
- Effect as noun: The breakfast I ate this morning had a negative *effect* on me.
- Effect as verb: He was able to *effect* change in his life after he became well again.

Among versus Between

When choosing between the words *between* and *among*, usually we would use *between* if it involved two choices, and *among* if it involved multiple choices. Here is an example:

I had to choose *between* purple and blue.

She distributed the ice cream *among* her four children.

This rule, however, isn't absolute. The word *between* can usually be used when talking about two or more things, if those things are distinct. For example:

He chose between vanilla, chocolate, and strawberry.

But if we are choosing among a group of things or people, or about items collectively, it is best to use *among*.

He chose among many ice cream flavors.

Amount versus Number

Amount is used with nouns that cannot be counted; *number* is used with nouns that can be counted. Here is an example:

No one knew the amount of bravery she was capable of.

The number of items on the list came to be twenty-seven.

Good versus Well

The word *good* is an adjective. We use the word *good* before nouns and after linking verbs. The word *well* is usually an adverb, although sometimes *well* can be an adjective when pertaining to someone's health.

Before a noun: Tina did a good job giving her speech in class today.

After linking verb: Tina's lunch smells good.

In the first example, we see that *good* is an adjective describing the word *job*. In the second example, the word *good* is an adjective to modify the subject *lunch*.

> Tina did well giving her speech in class today.

In the above example, *well* does not describe a noun; it answers the question *how did Tina do?* making *well* an adverb.

> Tina began to get well again after her surgery.

In the above example, we see *well* as an adjective pertaining to Tina and her health.

Bad versus Badly

Similar rules are applied to *bad* and *badly* just as in *good* and *well*. *Bad* is used to describe a noun or used after a linking verb. The word *badly* is an adverb that modifies an action verb. Let's look at the same example above using the word *bad* and *badly*:

> Before a noun: Tina did a bad job giving her speech in class today.

> After a linking verb: Tina's lunch smells bad.

> Badly as an adverb: Tina did badly giving her speech in class today.

Bring versus Take

The word *bring* implies carrying something toward the speaker, like *Please bring your pencils to class tomorrow*. The word *take* implies carrying something away from the speaker, like *Please take your pencils home with you tonight*.

Can versus May (Could versus Might)

In formal English, the word *may* is used to ask or grant permission, and the word *can* refers to ability or capability, like the following examples:

> May I go to the restroom before class starts?

> Can he ride his bicycle yet?

Keep these differences in mind while writing. With informal language, we often use *can* to ask permission, but in formal writing, it is more appropriate to use the word *may* when granting or asking for permission.

Farther versus Further

The word *farther* refers to a measurable or physical distance, like the following:

> How much farther is the walk to your house?

In the above context, the word *farther* is used because it is referring to a physical distance from one point to another.

The word *further* implies a metaphorical or figurative distance. *Further* may also mean "in addition to," like *I have nothing further to write*.

> We drifted further apart as the years went by.

Fewer versus Less

The word *fewer* is used with plural nouns and when discussing countable things. The word *less* is used with singular mass nouns. For example, we might have *fewer* coins, groceries, restaurants, or tablets, but we have *less* money, food, security, or light.

Hear versus Here

The word *hear* and *here* have distinctly different meanings, but they sound the same, so they are often misspelled. The word *hear* means to perceive with the ear, like *I hear the train coming this way*. The word *here* refers to a place or position, like *I put the money here a few seconds ago*.

i.e. versus e.g.

The abbreviation *i.e.* stands for "in other words." *I.e.* does not have to do with listing examples, but gives an alternate point of view of a statement, denoting the phrase "in other words."

The abbreviation *e.g.* stands for "for example." Use *e.g.* when listing one or more examples in your writing.

Learn versus Teach

The verb *learn* means to receive knowledge or a skill in a subject. The verb *teach* means to give knowledge or a skill to someone. Below are two examples of how to correctly use *learn* and *teach*.

Today, I learned how to count blocks in school.

Today, the teacher taught us how to count blocks in school.

Lie versus Lay

Excluding the definition of "to tell an untruth" for *lie*, the words *lay* and *lie* mean setting/reclining. The word *lay* requires a direct object. Here's an example:

Lay the book down on my desk please.

The word *book* in the sentence above is the direct object. If one were to lie down on the couch, it would be:

I want to lie down on the couch.

There is no direct object, so the verb *lie* is used.

What gets confusing between *lay* and *lie* is that *lay* is also a past tense of lie. In this case, we have:

Yesterday, Nina lay on the countertop and fell asleep.

Even more bizarre, the past tense of *lay* is *laid*. Therefore, we have:

Last week I laid the book down on your desk.

For the purposes of the present tense, remember that *lay* requires a direct object (you lay something down) and *lie* does not (you lie down by yourself).

Which versus That

Sometimes, it can be confusing when to use *which* or when to use *that* in a sentence. Basically, the word *that* is used for restrictive clauses (aka essential clauses). Restrictive clauses are clauses that restrict the information in another part of the sentence, so they cannot be taken out. Here's an example:

The door *that you broke* is being *fixed*.

The restrictive clause is in italics. If we took this information out, it would change the meaning of the sentence. It's a *very specific door* that is being fixed—the one *that you broke*. This information is pertinent to the sentence.

The word *which* is used for nonrestrictive clauses (aka nonessential clauses). This means that the clause beginning with *which* can be taken out of the sentence, and the information in the main clause will not be changed. Here are some examples:

I only got five hours of sleep last night, which isn't good.

Mangos, which are cheap, are my favorite food.

Notice in the second sentence, if we took out the middle clause *which are cheap*, mangos would still be the speaker's favorite food. Clauses that begin with *which* are almost always set apart by commas or preceded by commas.

Who versus Whom

The words *who* and *whom* serve two different purposes within a sentence. *Who* refers to the subject of a clause, which is the noun that is acting. *Whom* refers to the direct object of a clause, which is the noun that is having something done to it. Here are two examples using both *who* and *whom*:

Who left the door open last night?

Whom did you leave that letter with?

Let's answer these questions with the proper noun, *Marie. Marie left the door open last night.* In this sentence, we can see that *Marie* is the subject of the sentence. Since the *who* is referring to the subject of the sentence, the first example is correct. Let's answer the second question. *I left that letter with Marie.* Now, Marie is the *object* of the sentence. This sentence is correct because it uses *whom* to refer to the object of the sentence.

One trick is to replace the word *who* or *whom* with *she* or *her*. When using the word *who*, we can answer the question with *she, he*, or *they*. When using the word whom, we can answer the question with *her, him*, or them. Plugging the pronouns in is an easy way to tell if you've used the correct word:

She left the door open last night. (Who?)

I left the letter with *her*. (Whom?)

Notice again that the word *she* is the subject of the first sentence (so we use *who*), and the word *her* is the object of the second sentence (so we use *whom*).

HESI Grammar Practice Questions

1. Which of these is NOT a good way to improve writing style through grammar?
    a. Alternating among different sentence structures
    b. Using fewer words instead of unnecessary words
    c. Consistently using one-subject and one-verb sentences
    d. Writing in the active voice more than passive voice

2. Of the following statements, which is most accurate about topic sentences?
    a. They are always first in a paragraph.
    b. They are always last in a paragraph.
    c. They are only found once in every essay.
    d. They are explicit or may be implicit.

3. Which of the following is considered criteria for a good paragraph topic sentence?
    a. Clear
    b. Subtle
    c. Lengthy
    d. Ambiguous

4. "We don't go out as much because babysitters, gasoline, and parking is expensive." Which grammatical error does this sentence demonstrate?
    a. It contains a misplaced modifier.
    b. It lacks subject-verb agreement.
    c. It introduces a dangling participle.
    d. It does not have a grammar error.

5. Which of the following versions of a sentence has correct pronoun-antecedent agreement?
    a. Every student must consult their advisor first.
    b. All students must talk with their advisors first.
    c. All students must consult with his advisor first.
    d. Every student must consult their advisors first.

6. Which version of this sentence is grammatically correct?
    a. Give it to Shirley and I.
    b. Both Choices *C* and *D*.
    c. Give it to Shirley and me.
    d. Give it to me and Shirley.

7. What parts of speech are modified by adjectives?
    a. Verbs
    b. Nouns
    c. Pronouns
    d. Both Choices *B* and *C*

8. What part(s) of speech do adverbs modify?
    a. Verbs
    b. Adverbs
    c. Adjectives
    d. All of the above

9. What accurately reflects expert advice for beginning writers regarding topic sentences?
    a. They should use topic sentences in every two to three paragraphs.
    b. They should vary topic sentence positioning in paragraphs.
    c. They should include a topic sentence in every paragraph.
    d. They should make each topic sentence broad and general.

10. Being familiar with English words such as claustrophobia, *photophobia, arachnophobia, hydrophobia, acrophobia,* etc. could help a reader not knowing the origin determine that the Greek *phobos* means which of these?
    a. Love
    b. Fear
    c. Hate
    d. Know

11. Which of the following English words is derived from a Greek source?
    a. Move
    b. Motor
    c. Moron
    d. Mobile

12. Homophones are defined as which of these?
    a. They have the same sounds.
    b. They have the same spelling.
    c. They have the same meaning.
    d. They have the same roots.

13. The word *tear,* pronounced one way, means a drop of eye fluid; pronounced another way, it means to rip. What is this type of word called?
    a. A homograph
    b. A heteronym
    c. A homonym
    d. Both *A* and *B*

14. Which of these words is considered a plural?
    a. Cactus
    b. Bacteria
    c. Criterion
    d. Elf

15. Which of these words has an irregular plural that is the same as its singular form?
    a. Louse
    b. Goose
    c. Mouse
    d. Moose

16. Of the following words with irregular plurals, which one has a plural ending *most* different from those of the others?
    a. Ox
    b. Child
    c. Person
    d. Woman

17. Which of the following sentences uses the apostrophe(s) correctly?
    a. Please be sure to bring you're invitation to the event.
    b. All of your friends' invitations were sent the same day.
    c. All of your friends parked they're cars along the street.
    d. Who's car is parked on the street with it's lights on?

18. Of the following, which word is spelled correctly?
    a. Wierd
    b. Forfeit
    c. Beleive
    d. Concieve

19. Which of these words has the correct spelling?
    a. Insolent
    b. Irrelevent
    c. Independant
    d. Indispensible

20. Exceptions and variations in rules for capitalization are accurately reflected in which of these?
    a. *Congress* is capitalized and so is *Congressional.*
    b. *Constitution* is capitalized as well as *Constitutional.*
    c. *Caucasian* is capitalized, but *white,* referring to race, is not.
    d. *African-American* and *Black* as a race are both capitalized.

21. Which of the following statements is true about the Oxford comma?
    a. It is the first comma in a series of three or more items.
    b. It is the last comma in a series before *or,* or before *and.*
    c. It is any comma separating items in series of three or more.
    d. It is frequently omitted because it does not serve a purpose.

22. In the following sentence, which version has the correct punctuation?
    a. Delegates attended from Springfield; Illinois, Alamo; Tennessee, Moscow; Idaho, and other places.
    b. Delegates attended from Springfield Illinois, Alamo Tennessee, Moscow Idaho, and other places.
    c. Delegates attended from Springfield, Illinois; Alamo, Tennessee; Moscow, Idaho; and other places.
    d. Delegates attended from Springfield, Illinois, Alamo, Tennessee, Moscow, Idaho, and other places.

23. Of the following phrases, which correctly applies the rules for hyphenation?
    a. Finely-tuned
    b. Family owned
    c. Friendly looking
    d. Fraudulent-ID claim

24. What is the rule for using quotation marks with a quotation inside of a quotation?
    a. Single quotation marks around the outer quotation, double quotation marks around the inner one
    b. Double quotation marks to enclose the outer quotation and also to enclose the inner quotation
    c. Single quotation marks that enclose the outer quotation as well as the inner quotation
    d. Double quotation marks around the outer quotation, single quotation marks around the inner one

25. Which of the following phrases correctly uses apostrophes?
    a. Dennis and Pam's house
    b. Dennis's and Pam's house
    c. Dennis' and Pam's house
    d. Dennis's and Pam house

26. Which of these correctly applies the rule to make irregular plural nouns possessive?
    a. Geeses' honks
    b. Childrens' toys
    c. Teeths' enamel
    d. Women's room

27. Which of the following is a writing technique recommended for attaining sentence fluency?
    a. Varying the endings of sentences
    b. Making sentence lengths uniform
    c. Using consistent sentence rhythm
    d. Varying sentence structures used

28. Among elements of an effective paragraph, the element of coherence is reflected by which of these?
    a. Focus on one main point throughout
    b. The use of logical and verbal bridges
    c. A sentence identifying the main idea
    d. Data, examples, illustrations, analysis

29. What is the subject of the sentence: "Don't drink and drive."?
    a. Drink
    b. Drive
    c. Don't
    d. Understood *you*

30. The above sentence is an example of what type of sentence?
    a. Declarative
    b. Imperative
    c. Interrogative
    d. Exclamatory

31. *After*, *since*, and *whereas* are all examples of which of the following?
    a. Coordinate conjunctions
    b. Coordinate adjectives
    c. Demonstrative adjectives
    d. Subordinating conjunctions

32. All EXCEPT which of the following words or phrases are interjections?
    a. Good gracious
    b. Oh
    c. Ahh
    d. Running

33. An *independent clause* can be defined as which of the following?
    a. A sentence without a subject
    b. A sentence without a verb
    c. A sentence with a subject and verb that expresses a complete thought
    d. A sentence that is combined by a conjunction and preposition

34. *Beyond the wall*, *beside the car*, and *under the floor* are examples of which of the following?
    a. Prepositional phrases
    b. Occupational phrases
    c. Auxiliary phrases
    d. Dual phrases

35. *This, that*, and *those* can be used as both of which of the following?
    a. Demonstrative pronouns and adjectives
    b. Demonstrative adjectives and adverbs
    c. Clauses and compound sentences
    d. Prepositions and adjectives

36. The word *not* is which of the following?
    a. Adverb
    b. Adjective
    c. Noun
    d. Pronoun

37. A *complex sentence* can be defined as which of the following?
    a. A sentence that contains no prepositional phrases
    b. A sentence that contains an indefinite pronoun
    c. A sentence that contains two independent clauses
    d. A sentence that contains at least one independent clause and at least one dependent clause

38. Choose the sentence that contains a comma splice.
    a. The boys never met; they were strangers.
    b. The boys never met: they were strangers.
    c. The boys never met, they were strangers.
    d. The boys, never met; they were strangers.

39. Subjective case can also be called which of the following?
    a. Objective case
    b. Possessive case
    c. Adjective case
    d. Nominative case

40. The underlined portion of the following sentence contains an example of which grammatical convention?
    The woman behind you is my <u>mother</u>.
    a. Pronoun
    b. Predicate nominative
    c. Adjective
    d. Prepositional phrase

41. *Comparative* and *superlative* are types of which of the following?
    a. Nouns
    b. Adjectives and adverbs
    c. Verbs
    d. Pronouns

42. The underlined portion of the following sentence contains an example of which verb form?
    Sandy <u>will have finished</u> by the end of the second semester.
    a. Present
    b. Past perfect
    c. Future perfect
    d. Present progressive

43. Fill in the blank. Gerund phrases function as _____ in a sentence.
    a. Adjectives
    b. Adverbs
    c. Conjunctions
    d. Nouns

44. Which of the following sentences contains an example of passive voice?
    a. The poem was written by a student.
    b. The poem contained two metaphors and a simile.
    c. A student wrote the poem.
    d. A student decided to write a poem yesterday.

45. All EXCEPT which of the following words are examples of relative pronouns?
    a. Who
    b. Whom
    c. That
    d. These

46. Fill in the blank. A(n) _____ refers to whom or for whom the action of the verb is being done.
    a. Direct object
    b. Indirect object
    c. Subject object
    d. Object subject

47. "I like writing, playing soccer, and eating" is an example of which grammatical convention?
    a. Appositive
    b. Complement
    c. Verbal
    d. Parallelism

48. Transition words can be used for all EXCEPT which of the following purposes?
    a. To explain
    b. To compare
    c. As conjunctions
    d. To replace a verb

49. Run-on or fused sentences *must* contain two or more of which of the following?
    a. Dependent phrases
    b. Independent phrases
    c. Sentences with passive voice
    d. Independent clauses

50. Fill in the blank. Collective nouns are paired with _____ in a sentence.
    a. Collective verbs
    b. Singular verbs
    c. Singular nouns
    d. Plural verbs

Select the choice you think best fits the underlined part of the sentence. If the original is the best answer choice, then choose Choice A.

51. After getting a cat, Billy learned the meaning of take care of something other than himself.
    a. learned the meaning of
    b. learned what it meant to
    c. meant to learning the
    d. made to learn of the

52. A toothache does not always denote tooth decay or a cavity; sometimes it was the direct result of having a sinus infection.
    a. it was the direct
    b. it be the direct
    c. it directly was
    d. it is the direct

53. <u>Play baseball, swimming, and dancing</u> are three of Hannah's favorite ways to be active.
   a. Play baseball, swimming, and dancing
   b. Playing baseball; swimming; dancing;
   c. Playing baseball, to swim and to dance,
   d. Playing baseball, swimming, and dancing

54. <u>I was shocked by the sound of the blast muting</u> the television and went outside to see what happened.
   a. I was shocked by the sound of the blast muting
   b. I was shocked by the sound of the blast, muted
   c. Shocked at the sound of the blast, I muted
   d. The sound of the blast shocked me, muting

55. <u>The dog turned in a circle five times before its tail</u> went between its legs and it went to sleep.
   a. The dog turned in a circle five times before its tail
   b. For the dog, it turned around five times before its tail
   c. A dog's turning in a circle five times before its tail
   d. The dog turned in a circle five times before their tail

Answer Explanations

1. C: Good ways to improve writing style through grammatical choices include alternating among simple, complex, compound, and compound-complex sentence structures (Choice *A*) to prevent monotony and ensure variety; using fewer words when more words are unnecessary (Choice *B*); NOT writing all simple sentences with only one subject and one verb each (Choice *C*); and writing in the active voice more often than in the passive voice (Choice *D*). Active voice uses fewer words and also emphasizes action more strongly.

2. D: The topic sentence of a paragraph is often at or near the beginning, but not always, so Choice *A* is incorrect. Some topic sentences are at the ends of paragraphs but not always. Therefore, Choice *B* is incorrect. There is more than one topic sentence in an essay, especially if the essay is built on multiple paragraphs, so Choice *C* is incorrect. The topic sentence in a paragraph may be stated explicitly, or it may only be implied, requiring the reader to infer what the topic is rather than identify it as an overt statement. Thus, Choice *D* is correct.

3. A: Criteria for a good paragraph topic sentence include clarity, emphasis rather than subtlety, brevity rather than length, and straightforwardness rather than ambiguousness. Therefore, Choices *B, C,* and *D* are incorrect.

4. B: The sentence lacks subject-verb agreement. Three nouns require plural "are," not singular "is." A misplaced modifier (Choice *A*) is incorrectly positioned, modifying the wrong part. For example, in Groucho Marx's famous joke, "One morning I shot an elephant in my pajamas. How he got into my pajamas I don't know" (*Animal Crackers,* 1930), he refers in the second sentence to the misplaced modifier in the first. A dangling participle (Choice *C*) leaves a verb participle hanging by omitting the subject it describes; e.g. "Walking down the street, the house was on fire."

5. B: Choice *A* lacks pronoun-antecedent agreement: "Every student" is singular, but "their" is plural. Choice *B* correctly combines plural "All students" with plural "their advisors." Choice *C* has plural "All students" but singular "his advisor." Choice *D* has singular "Every student" but plural "their advisors."

6. B: When compounding subjects by adding nouns including proper nouns (names) to pronouns, the pronoun's form should not be changed by the addition. Since "Give it to me" is correct, not "Give it to I," we would not write "Give it to Shirley and I" (Choice *A*). "Shirley" and "me" are correct in either position in Choices *C* and *D*. "Give it to" requires an object. Only "me," "us," "him," "her," and "them" can be objects; "I," "we," "he," "she," and "they" are used as subjects but never as objects.

7. D: Adjectives modify nouns (Choice *B*) or pronouns (Choice *C*) by describing them. For example, in the phrase "a big, old, red house," the noun "house" is modified and described by the adjectives "big," "old," and "red." Adjectives do not modify verbs, adverbs do; therefore, Choice *A* is incorrect.

8. D: Adverbs modify verbs (Choice *A*), other adverbs (Choice *B*), or adjectives (Choice *C*). For example, in "She slept soundly," the verb is "slept" and the adverb modifying it is "soundly." In "He finished extremely quickly," the adverb "extremely" modifies the adverb "quickly." In "She was especially enthusiastic," the adverb "especially" modifies the adjective "enthusiastic."

9. C: Experts should advise students/beginning writers to include a topic sentence in every paragraph. Although professional writers do not always do this, beginners should, to learn how to write good topic sentences and paragraphs, rather than include a topic sentence in only every second or third paragraph, so Choice *A* is incorrect. Although experienced writers can also vary the positioning of topic sentences within paragraphs, experts advise new/learning writers to start paragraphs with topic sentences; therefore, Choice *B* is wrong. A topic sentence should be narrow and restricted, not broad and general; thus, Choice *D* is incorrect.

10. B: *Phobos* means "fear" in Greek. From it, English has derived the word *phobia,* meaning an abnormal or exaggerated fear and a multitude of other words ending in *-phobia,* whose beginnings specify the object of the fear, as in the examples given. Another ubiquitous English word part deriving from Greek is *phil* as a prefix or suffix, meaning love (Choice *A*), such as *philosophy, hydrophilic, philanthropist,* and *philharmonic.* The Greek word for hate (Choice *C*) is *miseo,* found in English words like *misogyny* and *misanthrope.* The Greek word meaning wise or knowledge (Choice *D*) is *sophos,* found in English words such as *sophisticated* and *philosophy.*

11. C: The English word *moron* is derived from the Greek *mor-* meaning dull or foolish. *Sophomore* also combines *soph* from Greek *sophos,* meaning wise, with *mor*—i.e. literally "wise fool." The words *move* (Choice *A*), *motor* (Choice *B*), *mobile* (Choice *D*), and many others are all derived from the Latin *mot-* or *mov-,* from the Latin words *movere,* to move and *motus,* motion.

12. A: Homophones are words that are pronounced the same way but are spelled differently and have different meanings. For example, *lax* and *lacks* are homophones. Words spelled the same (Choice *B*) but with different meanings are homographs. Words with the same meaning (Choice *C*) are synonyms, which are spelled and pronounced differently.

13. D: Words that are spelled the same way are homographs (Choice *A*); if they are pronounced differently, they are heteronyms (Choice *B*). The example given fits both definitions. But homonyms (Choice *C*) are spelled the same way (i.e. homographs) AND also pronounced the same way (i.e. homophones), NOT differently. Therefore, Choices *A* and *B* both correctly describe *tear,* but Choice *C* does not.

14. B: Bacteria is considered a plural word. The singular word for "bacteria" is "bacterium." Cactus, criterion, and elf are all considered singular words, making Choices *A, C,* and *D* incorrect.

15. D: *Moose* is both the singular and plural form of the word. Other words that do not change from singular to plural include *deer, fish,* and *sheep. Louse* (Choice *A*) has an irregular plural, but it is *lice,* not the same as the singular. *Goose* (Choice *B*) has the irregular plural *geese,* also not the same as the singular. *Mouse* (Choice *C*), like *louse,* has the irregular plural *mice,* also different from its singular form.

16. C: The irregular plural of *ox* (Choice *A*) is *oxen.* The irregular plural of *child* (Choice *B*) is *children.* The irregular plural of *woman* (Choice *D*) is *women.* These irregular plurals all end in *–en.* However, *person* (Choice *C*) has the irregular plural of *people,* which has a different ending than the others. It can also be pluralized as *persons;* but this is a regular plural, not an irregular one.

17. B: The plural possessive noun *friends'* is correctly punctuated with an apostrophe following the plural *-s* ending. *Friend's* would indicate a singular possessive noun, like something belonging to one friend. *Friends* would indicate a plural noun not possessing anything. In Choice *A,* the second-person possessive is *your,* NOT "you're," a contraction of "you are." In Choice *C,* the third-person plural possessive is *their,* NOT "they're," a contraction of "they are." There are two errors in Choice *D.* The first possessive is *whose,* NOT "who's," a contraction of "who is;" the second is *its,* NOT "it's," a contraction of "it is."

128

18. B: *Forfeit* is spelled correctly. Choice *A* is misspelled and should be *weird*. Choice *C* is misspelled and should be *believe*. Choice *D* is misspelled and should be *conceive*. Many people confuse the spellings of words with *ie* and *ei* combinations. Some rules that apply to most English words, with 22 exceptions, are: I before E except after C; and before L, P, T, or V; when sounding like *A* as in weight; when sounding like *I* as in height; or when an *ei* combination is formed by a prefix or a suffix.

19. A: *Insolent* is correctly spelled. Many people misspell words that sound the same but are spelled differently by confusing the vowels *a, e,* and *i*. For example, Choice *B* is correctly spelled *irrelevant;* Choice *C* is correctly spelled *independent;* and the correct spelling of Choice *D* is *indispensable.* Confusion is increased by these variations: Choices *B* and *C* sound the same but end with *-ant* and *-ent,* respectively; and while Choice *D* ends with *-able,* other words like *irrepressible* and *gullible* correctly end with *-ible,* which is incorrect in *indispensable.*

20. C: While terms like *Caucasian* and *African-American* are capitalized, the words *white* (Choice *C*) and *black* (Choice *D*) when referring to race should NOT be capitalized. While the name *Congress* is capitalized, the adjective *congressional* should NOT be capitalized (Choice *A*). Although the name of the U.S. *Constitution* is capitalized, the related adjective *constitutional* is NOT capitalized (Choice *B*).

21. B: The Oxford comma is the last comma following the last item in a series and preceding the word *or* or *and.* It is NOT the first (Choice *A*), or any comma separating items in a series (Choice *C*) other than the last. While it is true that many people omit this comma, it is NOT true that it serves no purpose (Choice *D*). It can prevent confusion when series include compound nouns.

22. C: A city and its state should always be separated by a comma. When items in a series contain internal commas, they should be separated by semicolons. City and state are never separated by a semicolon (Choice *A*). The city and its state are never named without punctuation between them (Choice *B*). The reason it is incorrect to use all commas, both between each city and its state and also between city-state pairs (Choice *D*), is obvious: some of the names used can refer to multiple places, causing serious confusion without different punctuation marks to identify them.

23. D: One rule for using hyphens is to clarify meaning: without the hyphen in this phrase, a reader could interpret it to mean that the claim is fraudulent; the hyphen makes it clear that it is the ID that is fraudulent. Another rule is that adverbs with *–ly* endings are not hyphenated, so (Choice *A*) should be *finely tuned.* However, an additional rule is that adjectives with *–ly* endings are hyphenated; hence Choice *B* should be *family-owned,* and Choice *C* should be *friendly-looking.*

24. D: The rule for writing a quotation with another quotation inside it is to use double quotation marks to enclose the outer quotation and use single quotation marks to enclose the inner quotation. Here is an example: "I don't think he will attend, because he said, 'I am extremely busy.'" The correct usage is reversed in Choice *A*. Choices *B* and *C* are incorrect, as this would not distinguish one quotation from the other.

25. A: When two people are named and both possess the same object, the apostrophe-*s* indicating possession should be placed ONLY after the second name, NOT after both names, making Choices *B* and *C* incorrect. It is also incorrect to use the apostrophe-*s* after the first name instead of the second (Choice *D*).

26. D: Irregular plurals that do not end in *–s* are always made possessive by adding apostrophe-*s.* A common error people make is to add *–s*-apostrophe instead of vice versa, as in the other three choices. *Geese* (Choice *A*), *children* (Choice *B*), and *teeth* (Choice *C*) are already plural, so adding an *s* before the apostrophe constitutes a double plural. Adding the *–s* after the apostrophe (i.e. *geese's, children's,* and *teeth's*) correctly makes these plurals possessive.

27. D: Some writing techniques recommended for attaining sentence fluency include varying the beginnings of sentences, making Choice *A* incorrect; varying sentence lengths rather than making them all uniform, making Choice *B* incorrect; varying sentence rhythms rather than consistently using the same rhythm, making Choice *C* incorrect; and varying sentence structures among simple, compound, complex, and compound-complex, making Choice *D* correct.

28. B: Four elements of an effective paragraph are unity, coherence, a topic sentence, and development. Focusing on one main point throughout (Choice *A*) the paragraph reflects the element of unity. Using logical and verbal bridges (Choice *B*) between/across sentences reflects the element of coherence. A sentence identifying the main idea (Choice *C*) of the paragraph reflects the element of a topic sentence. Citing data, giving examples, including illustrations, and analyzing (Choice *D*) the topic all reflect the element of developing the paragraph sufficiently.

29. D: Understood *you*. Choices *A, B,* and *C* are all verbs, so they cannot be the subject of the sentence. Choice *D* is the correct answer because commands often necessitate an understood *you.*

30. B: Imperative. Choice *A* is incorrect because declarative sentences are statements but not commands. Choice *C* is incorrect because interrogative sentences ask questions. Choice *D* is incorrect because exclamatory sentences express emotions. Since imperative sentences are commands, Choice *B* is the correct answer.

31. D: Subordinating conjunctions. Choices *B* and *C, coordinate adjectives* and *demonstrative adjectives,* are incorrect because *after, since,* and *whereas* are not adjectives. Choice *A, coordinate conjunctions,* is incorrect because coordinating conjunctions are placed between words when the writer wants to give equal emphasis to each word, like *and* or *but.* Choice *D* is correct because subordinating conjunctions such as *after, since,* and *whereas* are often used at the beginning of subordinating clauses.

32. D: Running. Choices *A, B,* and *C* are incorrect because interjections are used to express emotion. Choice *D* is correct because the word *running* is most commonly used as a verb or noun, not an interjection.

33. C: A sentence with a subject and verb that expresses a complete thought. Choices *A* and *B* are incorrect because they describe the characteristics of a phrase. Choice *D* is incorrect because a sentence cannot be combined by a preposition. Choice *C* is correct because an independent clause must contain a subject and verb and express a complete thought.

34. A: Prepositional phrases. Choices *B, C,* and *D* are not related. Choice *A* is correct because prepositional phrases are composed of prepositions and their objects.

35. A: Demonstrative pronouns and adjectives. Choices *C* and *D* are incorrect. Choice *B* is incorrect because the words are not adverbs. Choice *A* is correct because the words can be used as adjectives when they are used to describe nouns, or pronouns when they are used to replace nouns.

36. A: Adverb. Choices *B, C,* and *D* are incorrect. Choice *A* is correct because the word *not* can be used to modify an adjective, a verb, or another adverb.

37. D: A sentence that contains at least one independent clause and at least one dependent clause. Choices *A* and *B* are incorrect because the number of prepositional phrases or indefinite pronouns has no bearing on whether a sentence is considered complex. Choice *C* is incorrect because a sentence with two independent clauses is a compound sentence.

38. C: The boys never met, they were strangers. Choices *A* and *B* are not possibilities because they don't contain commas. Choice *D* is incorrect because a comma splice occurs when a comma is used to incorrectly join two independent clauses. Therefore, Choice *C* is correct.

39. D: Nominative case. Choices *A*, *B*, and *C* are incorrect. The objective case is commonly used as a form of noun or pronoun used in object complements, direct objects, subject of the infinitive, and object of a preposition. The possessive case is used to show possession. The adjective case does not occur within the English language. Therefore, Choice *D* is correct.

40. B: Predicate nominative. Choices *A*, *C*, and *D* are incorrect. The word *mother* is not a pronoun, adjective, or prepositional phrase. Choice *B* is correct because a predicate nominative occurs when a noun that refers to the subject appears in the predicate of the sentence.

41. B: Adjectives and adverbs. Choices *A*, *C*, and *D* are incorrect. There are no comparative or superlatives nouns, pronouns, or verbs. Therefore, Choice *B* is correct, since adjectives and adverbs are used to describe nouns or modify adjectives, verbs, and other adverbs.

42. C: Future perfect. Choices *A*, *B*, and *D* are incorrect. Choice *C* is correct because the word *will* in the verb phrase *will have finished* denotes that the action will occur in the future.

43. D: Nouns. Choices *A*, *B*, and *C* are incorrect. Choice *D* is correct because gerund phrases contain gerunds, which are verbs that function as nouns in a sentence.

44. A: The poem was written by a student. Choices *B*, *C*, and *D* are incorrect. Choice *A* is correct because passive voice occurs when the subject is acted upon by the verb.

45. D: These. Choices *A*, *B*, and *C* are relative pronouns. Relative pronouns are used to join a clause or phrase to a noun or pronoun. Therefore, Choice *D* is the correct answer.

46. B: Indirect object. Choices *C* and *D* are not related. Choice *A* is incorrect because a direct object receives the action of the verb. Choice *B* is correct because an indirect object refers to whom or for whom the action of the verb is being done.

47. D: Parallelism. Choices *A*, *B*, and *C* are all unrelated. Choice *D* is correct because parallelism refers to the state of being the same or congruent. The present participles *writing, playing,* and *eating* are congruent parts of speech within a list and are thus parallel.

48. D: To replace a verb. Choices *A*, *B*, and *C* are incorrect. Choice *D* is correct. Transition words cannot be used to replace a verb.

49. D: Independent clauses. Choices *A* and *B* are unrelated and incorrect. Choice *C* is incorrect because passive voice has no bearing on whether a sentence is a run-on or a fused sentence. Choice *D* is correct because a run-on or fused sentence occurs when two independent clauses are joined incorrectly.

50. B: Collective nouns, such as team, family, and band, describe a group of individuals, animals, or things. They are paired with singular verbs. For example, "the family moved to Greece." Collective verbs, Choice *A,* do not exist. Collective nouns are not necessarily paired with singular nouns in the subject of a sentence, and are not paired with plural verbs, so Choices *C* and *D* are incorrect.

51. B: The correct answer is Choice *B*: "Billy learned what it meant to take care of something other than himself." Choice *A* is awkwardly worded and doesn't flow with the rest of the sentence. Choice *C*, "meant to learning" is also incorrect because it is missing a "to" after the phrase, and the word "learning" is also in the wrong verb form. Choice *D* is also worded awkwardly and thus the latter part of the sentence is unclear with this phrase.

52. D: The sentence should read: "sometimes it is the direct result of having a sinus infection." Choice *A* is incorrect because "was" is in past tense, and the rest of the sentence is in present tense. Choice *B* is incorrect because "it be" is not proper subject/verb agreement. "Be" should be conjugated to "is" as a be-verb. Finally, Choice *C* is incorrect; we have a past tense "was" which is incorrect, we are missing the article "the," and it is poorly worded.

53. D: Choice *D* is the best answer choice because the gerunds are all in parallel structure: "Playing baseball, swimming, and dancing." Choice *A* is incorrect because "Play baseball" does not match the parallel structure of the other two gerunds. Choice *B* is incorrect because the answer uses semicolons instead of commas, which is incorrect. Semicolons are used to separate independent clauses. Choice *C* is incorrect because "to swim" and "to dance" eschew parallel structure.

54. C: The correct answer is Choice *C*: "Shocked at the sound of the blast, I muted the television and went outside to see what happened." Choice *A* is incorrect because we're not sure if it is the "I" that's doing the muting or the blast. Choice *B* has incorrect sentence structure. We have "I was shocked" and that carries over to "I was muted," which is incorrect. We need someone doing the muting without the helping verb. Choice *D* is incorrect; we don't have a proper subject to go with the verb "muting." "Me muting" is not correct. Right now, it's the "sound" that's doing the muting, and this is incorrect.

55. A: Choice *A* is the best answer because it is the most straightforward. Choice *B* adds "For the dog, it turned around," which makes the sentence more confusing than the simple, "The dog turned in a circle." Choice *C* is incorrect because "A dog turned" is clearer subject/verb agreement than "A dog's turning," which does not match the other verb tense. Choice *D* has incorrect pronoun agreement; "their" should be "its" because there is only one dog.

Biology

Biology Basics

Atoms are the smallest units of all matter and make up all chemical elements. They each have three parts: protons, neutrons, and electrons. **Protons** are found in the nucleus of an atom and have a positive electric charge. They have a mass of about one atomic mass unit. The number of protons in an element is referred to as the element's *atomic number*. Each element has a unique number of protons and therefore its own unique atomic number. **Neutrons** are also found in the nucleus of atoms. These subatomic particles have a neutral charge, meaning that they do not have a positive or negative electric charge. Their mass is slightly larger than that of a proton. Together with protons, they are referred to as the *nucleons of an atom*. The *atomic mass number* of an atom is equal to the sum of the protons and neutrons in the atom. **Electrons** have a negative charge and are the smallest of the subatomic particles. They are located outside the nucleus in *orbitals*, which are shells that surround the nucleus. If an atom has an overall neutral charge, it has an equal number of electrons and protons. If it has more protons than electrons or vice versa, it becomes an *ion*. When there are more protons than electrons, the atom is a positively-charged ion, or *cation*. When there are more electrons than protons, the atom is a negatively-charged ion, or *anion*.

The location of electrons within an atom is more complicated than the locations of protons and neutrons. Within the orbitals, electrons are always moving. They can spin very fast and move upward, downward, and sideways. There are many different levels of orbitals around the atomic nucleus, and each orbital has a different capacity for electrons. The electrons in the orbitals closest to the nucleus are more tightly bound to the nucleus of the atom. There are three main characteristics that describe each orbital. The first is the principle quantum number, which describes the size of the orbital. The second is the angular momentum quantum number, which describes the shape of the orbital. The third is the magnetic quantum number, which describes the orientation of the orbital in space.

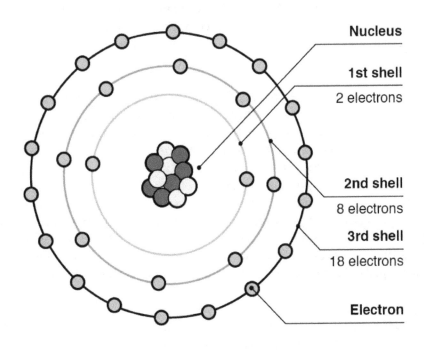

Nucleus

1st shell

2 electrons

2nd shell

8 electrons

3rd shell

18 electrons

Electron

Another important characteristic of electrons is their ability to form covalent bonds with other atoms to form molecules. A **covalent bond** is a chemical bond that forms when two atoms share the same pair or pairs of electrons. There is a stable balance of attraction and repulsion between the two atoms. There are several types of covalent bonds. **Sigma bonds** are the strongest type of covalent bond and involve the head-on overlapping of electron orbitals from two different atoms. **Pi bonds** are a little weaker and involve the lateral overlapping of certain orbitals. While single bonds between atoms, such as between carbon and hydrogen, are generally sigma bonds, double bonds, such as when carbon is double-bonded to an oxygen atom, are usually one sigma bond and one pi bond.

Water

The universe is composed completely of matter. **Matter** is any material or object that takes up space and has a mass. Although there is an endless variety of items found in the universe, there are only about one hundred elements, or individual substances, that make up all matter. These *elements* are different types of atoms and are the smallest units that anything can be broken down into while still retaining the properties of the original substance. Different elements can link together to form compounds, or molecules. Hydrogen and oxygen are two examples of elements, and when they bond together, they form water molecules. Matter can be found in three different states: gas, liquid, or solid.

Gases

Gases have three main distinct properties. The first is that they are easy to compress. When a gas is compressed, the space between the molecules decreases, and the frequency of collisions between them increases. The second property is that they do not have a fixed volume or shape. They expand to fill large containers or compress down to fit into smaller containers. When they are in large containers, the gas molecules can float around at high speeds and collide with each other, which allows them to fill the entire container uniformly. Therefore, the volume of a gas is generally equal to the volume of its container. The third distinct property of a gas is that it occupies more space than the liquid or solid from which it was formed. One gram of solid CO_2, also known as *dry ice,* has a volume of 0.641 milliliters. The same amount of CO_2 in a gaseous state has a volume of 556 milliliters. Steam engines use water in this capacity to do work. When water boils inside the steam engine, it becomes steam, or water vapor. As the steam increases in volume and escapes its container, it is used to make the engine run.

Liquids

A *liquid* is an intermediate state between gases and solids. It has an exact volume due to the attraction of its molecules to each other and molds to the shape of the part of the container that it is in. Although liquid molecules are closer together than gas molecules, they still move quickly within the container they are in. Liquids cannot be compressed, but their molecules slide over each other easily when poured out of a container. The attraction between liquid molecules, known as *cohesion,* also causes liquids to have surface tension. They stick together and form a thin skin of particles with an extra strong bond between them. As long as these bonds remain undisturbed, the surface becomes quite strong and can even support the weight of an insect such as a water skipper. Another property of liquids is adhesion, which is when different types of particles are attracted to each other. When liquids are in a container, they are drawn up above the surface level of the liquid around the edges. The liquid molecules that are in contact with the container are pulled up by their extra attraction to the particles of the container.

Solids

Unlike gases and liquids, *solids* have a definitive shape. They are similar to liquids in that they also have a definitive volume and cannot be compressed. The molecules are packed together tightly, which does not

134

allow for movement within the substance. There are two types of solids: crystalline and amorphous. *Crystalline solids* have atoms or molecules arranged in a specific order or symmetrical pattern throughout the entire solid. This symmetry makes all of the bonds within the crystal of equal strength, and when they are broken apart, the pieces have straight edges. Minerals are all crystalline solids. *Amorphous solids*, on the other hand, do not have repeating structures or symmetry. Their components are heterogeneous, so they often melt gradually over a range of temperatures. They do not break evenly and often have curved edges. Examples of amorphous solids are glass, rubber, and most plastics.

Matter can change between a gas, liquid, and solid. When these changes occur, the change is physical and does not affect the chemical properties or makeup of the substance. Environmental changes, such as temperature or pressure changes, can cause one state of matter to convert to another state of matter. For example, in very hot temperatures, solids can melt and become a liquid, such as when ice melts into liquid water, or sublimate and become a gas, such as when dry ice becomes gaseous carbon dioxide. Liquids can evaporate and become a gas, such as when liquid water turns into water vapor. In very cold temperatures, gases can depose and become a solid, such as when water vapor becomes icy frost on a windshield, or condense and become a liquid, such as when water vapor becomes dew on grass. Liquids can freeze and become a solid, such as when liquid water freezes and becomes ice.

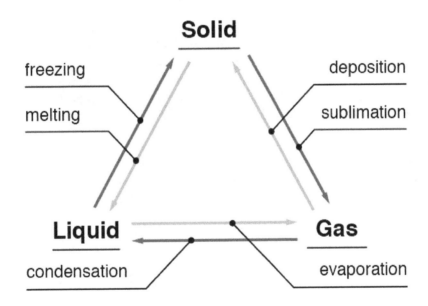

Biologic Molecules

There are six major elements found in most biological molecules: carbon, hydrogen, oxygen, nitrogen, sulfur, and phosphorus. These elements link together to make up the basic macromolecules of the biological system, which are lipids, carbohydrates, nucleic acids, and proteins. Most of these molecules use carbon as their backbone because of its ability to bond four different atoms. Each type of macromolecule has a specific structure and important function for living organisms.

Lipids
Lipids are made up of hydrocarbon chains, which are large molecules with hydrogen atoms attached to a long carbon backbone. These biological molecules are characterized as *hydrophobic* because their

structure does not allow them to form bonds with water. When mixed together, the water molecules bond to each other and exclude the lipids. There are three main types of lipids: triglycerides, phospholipids, and steroids.

Triglycerides are made up of one glycerol molecule attached to three fatty acid molecules. **Glycerols** are three-carbon atom chains with one hydroxyl group attached to each carbon atom. Fatty acids are hydrocarbon chains with a backbone of sixteen to eighteen carbon atoms and a double-bonded oxygen molecule. Triglycerides have three main functions for living organisms. They are a source of energy when carbohydrates are not available, they help with the absorption of certain vitamins, and they help insulate the body and maintain normal core temperature.

Phospholipid molecules have two fatty acid molecules bonded to one glycerol molecule, with the glycerol molecules having a phosphate group attached to it. The phosphate group has an overall negative charge, which makes that end of the molecule *hydrophilic*, meaning that it can bond with water molecules. Since the fatty acid tails of phospholipids are hydrophobic, these molecules are left with the unique characteristic of having different affinities on each of their ends. When mixed with water, phospholipids create *bilayers*, which are double rows of molecules with the hydrophobic ends on the inside facing each other and the hydrophilic ends on the outside, shielding the hydrophobic ends from the water molecules. Cells are protected by phospholipid bilayer cell membranes. This allows them to mix with aqueous solutions while also protecting their inner contents.

Steroids have a more complex structure than the other types of lipids. They are made up of four fused carbon rings. Different types of steroids are defined by the different chemical groups that attach to the carbon rings. Steroids are often mixed into phospholipid bilayers to help maintain the structure of the cell membrane and aid in cell signaling from these positions. They are also essential for regulation of metabolism and immune responses, among other biological processes.

Triglyceride

glycerol

H_2C — C — CH_2
       | | |
       H
       O   O   O

O   O   O

fatty
acids
(x 3)

Phospholipid

phosphate

NH$_3$

O
|
O — P — O$^-$
|
O

glycerol

H_2C — C — CH_2
       | | |
       H
       O   O

O   O

fatty
acids
(x 3)

Steroid

OH

H_2C

H_3C H_3C

4 fused
hydrocarbon
rings

CH_3

CH_3

136

Carbohydrates

Carbohydrates are made up of sugar molecules. Monomers are small molecules, and polymers are larger molecules that consist of repeating monomers. The smallest sugar molecule, or monomer, has the chemical formula of CH_2O. Monosaccharides can be made up of one of these small molecules or a multiple of this formula (such as $C_2H_4O_2$). Polysaccharides consist of repeating monosaccharides in lengths of a few hundred to a few thousand linked together. Monosaccharides are broken down by living organisms to extract energy from the sugar molecules for immediate consumption. Glucose is a common monosaccharide used by the body as a primary energy source and which can be metabolized immediately. The more complex structure of polysaccharides allows them to have a more long-term use. They can be stored and broken down later for energy. Glycogen is a molecule that consists of 1700 to 600,000 glucose units linked together. It is not soluble in water and can be stored for long periods of time. If necessary, the glycogen molecule can be broken up into single glucose molecules in order to provide energy for the body. Polysaccharides also form structurally strong materials, such as chitin, which makes up the exoskeleton of many insects, and cellulose, which is the material that surrounds plant cells.

Nucleic Acids

Nucleotides are made up of a five-carbon sugar molecule with a nitrogen-containing base and one or more phosphate groups attached to it. **Nucleic acids** are polymers of nucleotides, or polynucleotides. There are two main types of nucleic acids: **deoxyribonucleic acid (DNA)** and **ribonucleic acid (RNA)**. DNA is a double strand of nucleotides that are linked together and folded into a helical structure. Each strand is made up of four nucleotides, or bases: adenine, thymine, cytosine, and guanine. The adenine bases only pair with thymine on the opposite strand, and the cytosine bases only pair with guanine on the opposite strand. It is the links between these base pairs that create the helical structure of double-stranded DNA. DNA is in charge of long-term storage of genetic information that can be passed on to subsequent generations. It also contains instructions for constructing other components of the cell. RNA, on the other hand, is a single-stranded structure of nucleotides that is responsible for directing the construction of proteins within the cell. RNA is made up of three of the same nucleotides as DNA, but instead of thymine, adenine pairs with the base uracil.

Proteins

Proteins are made from a set of twenty amino acids that are linked together linearly, without branching. The amino acids have peptide bonds between them and form polypeptides. These polypeptide molecules coil up, either individually or as multiple molecules linked together, and form larger biological molecules, which are called *proteins*. Proteins have four distinct layers of structure. The primary structure consists of the sequence of amino acids. The secondary structure consists of the folds and coils formed by the hydrogen bonding that occurs between the atoms of the polypeptide backbone.

The tertiary structure consists of the shape of the molecule, which comes from the interactions of the side chains that are linked to the polypeptide backbone. Lastly, the quaternary structure consists of the overall shape that the protein takes on when it is made up of two or more polypeptide chains. Proteins have many vital roles in living organisms. They help maintain and repair body tissue, provide a source of energy, form antibodies to aid the immune system, and are a large component in transporting molecules within the body, among many other functions.

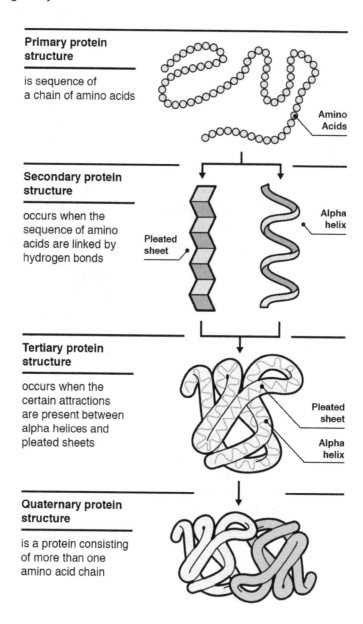

Metabolism

Metabolism includes all of the chemical reactions that take place within the cells of a living organism and provides energy and nutrition for survival of the organism. These reactions are vital for movement, growth, development, and reproduction. Organisms extract energy from materials in their surrounding environment to carry out these chemical reactions. In *catabolic reactions*, complex molecules are broken down into smaller, simpler molecules and more energy is released with the products than was required to start the reaction. Contrastingly, in *anabolic reactions*, simpler molecules are combined and built up into larger, more complex molecules, which requires a greater input of energy at the start of the reaction. The energy that is released by catabolic pathways is most often used to drive anabolic pathways forward. Cell metabolism is dictated by the first law of thermodynamics, which states that energy can be transformed but cannot be created or destroyed. Metabolic reactions can also be classified as either endergonic or exergonic. *Endergonic reactions* require input of energy, and the products contain more free energy than the sum of the reactants. *Exergonic reactions* release energy, so their products have less free energy than the sum of the reactants. They are said to occur spontaneously.

Adenosine triphosphate (ATP) is an essential molecule in metabolic pathways. It is created when nutrients, especially sugars, are broken down and cells use it as a direct source of energy. Once it is created, it provides energy for anabolic reactions and for movement of living organisms. One glucose molecule can produce approximately thirty ATP molecules in the presence of oxygen. Without oxygen, however, one glucose molecule only produces two ATP molecules. ATP also plays a role in cell signaling. It can keep track of how much ATP is present in the cell and signals whether nutrients should be stored and broken down later or if they should be broken down immediately to produce more ATP right away.

Enzymes are often an essential part of metabolic pathways. They are responsible for speeding up the rate of the metabolic reactions. Many biological reactions would not sustain life without enzymatic involvement. It is important to note that they do not change the amount of energy that is used up or released in the reaction; they only cause the reaction to start and reach completion more quickly. Each enzyme also only works on the specific reaction it was created for. Enzymes fit snugly into the substrate of the reactants of that specific reaction. Without the tight fit to activate the enzyme, the speed of the reaction will not increase.

The Cell

All living organisms are made up cells. **Cells** are considered the basic functional unit of organisms and the smallest unit of matter that is living. Most organisms are multicellular, which means that they are made up of more than one cell and often they are made up of a variety of different types of cells. Cells contain organelles, which are the little working parts of the cell, responsible for specific functions that keep the cell and organism alive.

Plant and animal cells have many of the same organelles but also have some unique traits that distinguish them from each other. Plants contain a cell wall, while animal cells are only surrounded by a phospholipid plasma membrane. The cell wall is made up of strong, fibrous polysaccharides and proteins. It protects the cell from mechanical damage and maintains the cell's shape. Inside the cell wall, plant cells also have plasma membrane. The plasma membrane of both plant and animal cells is made up of two layers of phospholipids, which have a hydrophilic head and hydrophobic tails. The tails converge towards each other on the inside of the bilayer, while the heads face the interior of the cell and the exterior environment. Microvilli are protrusions of the cell membrane that are only found in animal cells. They increase the surface area and aid in absorption, secretion, and cellular adhesion. Chloroplasts are also only found in plant cells. They are responsible for photosynthesis, which is how plants convert sunlight into chemical energy.

The list below describes major organelles that are found in both plant and animal cells:

- Nucleus: The nucleus contains the DNA of the cell, which has all of the cells' hereditary information passed down from parent cells. DNA and protein are wrapped together into chromatin within the nucleus. The nucleus is surrounded by a double membrane called the nuclear envelope.

- Endoplasmic Reticulum (ER): The ER is a network of tubules and membranous sacs that are responsible for the metabolic and synthetic activities of the cell, including synthesis of membranes. Rough ER has ribosomes attached to it while smooth ER does not.

- Mitochondrion: The mitochondrion is essential for maintaining regular cell function and is known as the powerhouse of the cell. It is where cellular respiration occurs and where most of the cell's ATP is generated.

- Golgi Apparatus: The Golgi Apparatus is where cell products are synthesized, modified, sorted, and secreted out of the cell.

- Ribosomes: Ribosomes make up a complex that produces proteins within the cell. They can be free in the cytosol or bound to the ER.

Cellular Respiration

Cellular respiration in multicellular organisms occurs in the mitochondria. It is a set of reactions that converts energy from nutrients to ATP and can either use oxygen in the process, which is called aerobic respiration, or not, which is called anaerobic respiration.

Aerobic respiration has two main parts, which are the citric acid cycle, also known as Krebs cycle, and oxidative phosphorylation. Glucose is a commonly found molecule that is used for energy production within the cell. Before the citric acid cycle can begin, the process of glycolysis converts glucose into two pyruvate molecules. Pyruvate enters the mitochondrion, is oxidized, and then is converted to a compound called acetyl CoA. There are eight steps in the citric acid cycle that start with acetyl CoA and convert it to oxaloacetate and NADH. The oxaloacetate continues in the citric acid cycle and the NADH molecule moves on to the oxidative phosphorylation part of cellular respiration. Oxidative phosphorylation has two main steps, which are the electron transport chain and chemiosmosis. The mitochondrial membrane has four protein complexes within it that help to transport electrons through the inner mitochondrial matrix. Electrons and protons are removed from NADH and $FADH_2$ and then transported along these and other membrane complexes.

Protons are pumped across the inner membrane, which creates a gradient to draw electrons to the intermembrane complexes. Two mobile electron carriers, ubiquinone and cytochrome C, are also located in the inner mitochondrial membrane. At the end of these electron transport chains, the electrons are accepted by O_2 molecules and water is formed with the addition of two hydrogen atoms. Chemiosmosis occurs in an ATP synthase complex that is located next to the four electron transport complexes. As the complex pumps protons from the intermembrane space to the mitochondrial matrix, ADP molecules become phosphorylated and ATP molecules are generated.

Approximately four to six ATP molecules are generated during glycolysis and the citric acid cycle and twenty-six to twenty-eight ATP molecules are generated during oxidative phosphorylation, which makes the total number of ATP molecules generated during aerobic cellular respiration approximately thirty to thirty-two.

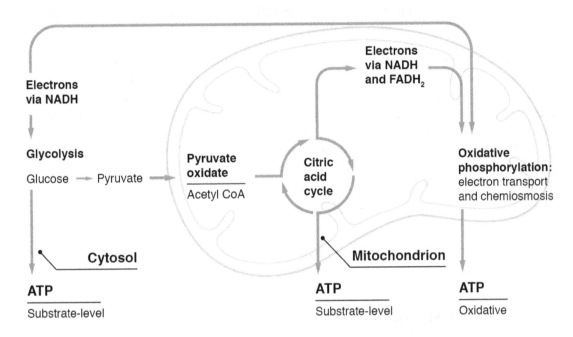

Since not all environments are oxygen-rich, some organisms must find alternate ways to extract energy from nutrients. The process of anaerobic respiration is similar to that of aerobic respiration in that protons and electrons are removed from nutrient molecules and are passed down an electron transport chain, with the end result being ATP synthesis. However, instead of the electrons being accepted by oxygen molecules at the end of the electron transport chain, they are accepted by either sulfate or nitrate molecules. Anaerobic respiration is mostly used by unicellular organisms, or prokaryotic organisms.

Photosynthesis

Photosynthesis is a set of reactions that occur to convert light energy into chemical energy. The chemical energy is then stored as sugar and other organic molecules inside the organism or plant. Within plants, the photosynthetic process takes place within chloroplasts. The two stages of photosynthesis are the light reactions and the Calvin cycle. Within chloroplasts, there are membranous sacs called *thylakoids* and within the thylakoids are a green pigment called chlorophyll. The light reactions take place in the chlorophyll. The Calvin cycle takes place in the *stroma*, or inner space, or the chloroplasts.

During the light reactions, light energy is absorbed by chlorophyll. First, a light-harvesting complex, called photosystem II (PS II), absorbs photons from light that enters the chlorophyll and then passes it onto a reaction-center complex. Once the photon enters the reaction-center complex, it causes a special pair of chlorophyll *a* molecules to release an electron. The electron is accepted by a primary electron acceptor molecule, while at the same time, a water molecule is dissociated into two hydrogen atoms, one oxygen atom, and two electrons. These electrons are transferred to the chlorophyll *a* molecules that just lost their electrons. The electrons that were released from the chlorophyll *a* molecules move down an electron transport chain using an electron carrier, called *plastoquinone*, a cytochrome complex, and a protein, called *plastocyanin*. At the end of the chain, the electrons reach another light-harvesting complex, called photosystem I (PS I). While in the cytochrome complex, the electrons cause protons to be pumped into the thylakoid space, which in turn provides energy for ATP molecules to be produced. A primary electron acceptor molecule accepts the electrons that are released from PS I and then passes them onto another electron transport chain, which includes the protein ferredoxin. At the end of the light reactions, electrons are transferred from ferredoxin to NADP+, producing NADPH. The ATP and NADPH that are produced through the light reactions are used as energy to drive the Calvin cycle forward.

The three phases of the **Calvin cycle** are carbon fixation, reduction, and regeneration of the CO_2 acceptor. Carbon fixation occurs when CO_2 is introduced into the cycle and attaches to a five-carbon sugar, called ribulose bisphosphate (RuBP). A six-carbon sugar is split into two three-carbon sugar molecules, known as 3-phosphoglycerate. Next, during the reduction phase, an ATP molecule loses a phosphate group and becomes ADP. The phosphate group attaches to the 3-phosphoglycerate molecule, making it 1,3-bisphosphate. Then, an NADPH molecule donates two electrons to this new molecule, causing it to lose a phosphate group and become glyceraldehyde 3-phosphate (G3P), a sugar molecule. At the end of the cycle, one G3P molecule exits the cycle and is used by the plant for energy.

Five other G3P molecules continue in the cycle to regenerate RuBP molecules, which are the CO_2 acceptors of the cycle. When every photon has been used up, three RuBP molecules are formed from the rearrangement of five G3P molecules and wait for the cycle to start again. It takes three turns of the cycle and three CO_2 molecules entering the cycle to generate just one G3P molecule.

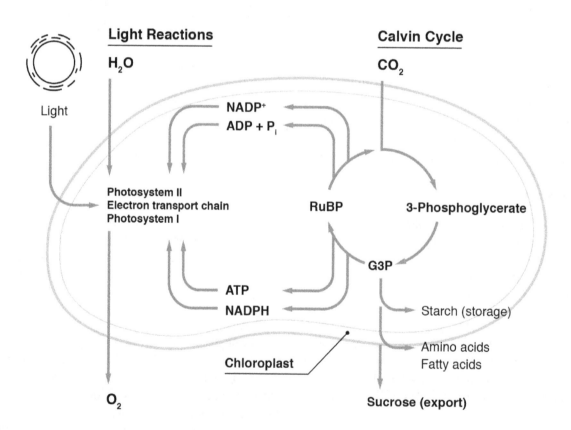

Cellular Reproduction

Cellular reproduction is the process that cells follow to make new cells with the same or similar contents as themselves. This process is an essential part of an organism's life. It allows for the organism to grow larger itself, and as it ages, it allows for replacement of dying and damaged cells. The process of cellular reproduction must be accurate and precise. Otherwise, the new cells that are produced will not be able to perform the same functions as the original cell. Mutations can occur in the offspring, which can cause anywhere from minor to severe problems. The two types of cellular reproduction that organisms can use are mitosis or meiosis. Mitosis produces daughter cells that are identical to the parent cell and is often referred to as asexual reproduction. Meiosis has two stages of cell division and produces daughter cells that have a combination of traits from their two parents. It is often referred to as sexual reproduction. Humans reproduce by meiosis. During this process, the sperm, the male germ cell, and the egg, the female germ cell, combine and form a parent cell that contains both of their sets of chromosomes. This parent cell then divides into four daughter cells, each with a unique set of traits that came from both of their parents.

In both processes, the most important part of the cell that is copied is the cell's DNA. It contains all of the genetic information for the cell, which leads to its traits and capabilities. Some parts of the cell are copied exactly during cellular reproduction, such as DNA. However, certain other cellular components are synthesized within the new cell after reproduction is complete using the new DNA. For example, the endoplasmic reticulum is broken down during the cell cycle and then newly synthesized after cell division.

Genetics

Humans carry their genetic information on structures called **chromosomes**. Chromosomes are string-like structures made up of nucleic acids and proteins. During the process of reproduction, each parent contributes a gamete that contains twenty-three chromosomes to the intermediate diploid cell. This diploid cell, which contains forty-six chromosomes, replicates itself to produce two diploid cells. These two diploid cells each then split into cells and randomly divide the chromosomes so that each of the four resulting cells contains only twenty-three chromosomes, as each parent gamete does.

Each of the twenty-three chromosomes has between a few hundred and a few thousand genes on it. Each gene contains information about a specific trait that is inherited by the offspring from one of the parents. Genes are made up of sequences of DNA that encode proteins and start pathways to express the phenotype that they control. Every gene has two alleles, or variations—one inherited from each parent. In most genes, one allele has a more dominant phenotype than the other allele. This means that when both alleles are present on a gene, the dominant phenotype will always be expressed over the recessive phenotype. The recessive phenotype would only be expressed when both alleles present were recessive.

Some alleles can have codominance or incomplete dominance. *Codominance* occurs when both alleles are expressed equally when they are both present. For example, the hair color of cows can be red or white, but when one allele for each hair color is present, their hair is a mix of red and white, not pink. *Incomplete dominance* occurs when the presence of two different alleles creates a third phenotype. For example, some flowers can be red or white when the alleles are in duplicate, but when one of each allele is present, the flowers are pink.

Mendel's Laws of Heredity

Gregor Mendel was a monk who came up with one of the first models of inheritance in the 1860s. He is often referred to as the father of genetics. At the time, his theories were largely criticized because biologists did not believe that these ideas could be generally applicable and could also not apply to different species. They were later rediscovered in the early 1900s and given more credence by a group of European scientists. Mendel's original ideas have since been combined with other theories of inheritance to develop the ideas that are studied today.

Between 1856 and 1863, Gregor Mendel experimented with about five thousand pea plants in his garden that had different color flowers to test his theories of inheritance. He crossed purebred white flower and purple flower pea plants and found that the results were not a blend of the two flowers; they were instead all purple flowers. When he then fertilized this second generation of purple flowers with itself, both white flowers and purple flowers were produced, in a ratio of one to three. Although he used different terms at the time, he proposed that the color trait for the flowers was regulated by a gene, which he called a *factor,* and that there were two alleles, which he called *forms,* for each gene. For each gene, one allele was inherited from each parent. The results of these experiments allowed him to come up with his Principles of Heredity.

There are two main laws that Mendel developed after seeing the results of his experiments. The first law is the **Law of Segregation**, which states that each trait has two versions that can be inherited. In the parent cells, the allele pairs of each gene separate, or segregate, randomly during gamete production. Each gamete then carries only one allele with it for reproduction. During the process of reproduction, the gamete from each parent contributes its single allele to the daughter cell. The second law is the Law of Independent Assortment, which states that the alleles for different traits are not linked to one another and are inherited independently. It emphasizes that if a daughter cell selects allele A for gene 1, it does not also automatically select allele A for gene 2. The allele for gene 2 is selected in a separate, random manner.

Mendel theorized one more law, called the **Law of Dominance**, which has to do with the expression of a genotype but not with the inheritance of a trait. When he crossed the purple flower and white flower pea plants, he realized that the purple flowers were expressed at a greater ratio than the white flower pea plants. He hypothesized that certain gene alleles had a stronger outcome on the phenotype that was expressed. If a gene had two of the same allele, the phenotype associated with that allele was expressed. If a gene had two different alleles, the phenotype was determined by the dominant allele, and the other allele, the recessive allele, had no effect on the phenotype.

DNA

DNA is made up of two polynucleotide strands that are linked together and twisted into a double-helix structure. The polynucleotide strands are made up a chain of nucleotides made from four nitrogenous bases, which are adenine, thymine, guanine, and cytosine. Across the two strands, adenine and thymine are paired together, and guanine and cytosine are paired together. This allows for a tight helix to form based on their molecular configurations. DNA contains all of the genetic information of a living organism and provides the protein encoding information on genes. Chromosome replication and cell division start with DNA replication. It is the first step in passing genetic information to subsequent generations. During replication, the double-helix DNA is untwisted and separated. Each strand is replicated and then linked to one of the original strands to form two new DNA molecules.

Sometimes, there are errors made in the DNA sequence that codes for a specific gene, causing genetic mutations. If the sequence alteration was originally in the parent gene, it is considered hereditary. If it was developed during the replication process, it is classified as an acquired mutation. Some mutations can cause major phenotypic differences, resulting in developmental problems, while others do not affect development at all. Although they are not very common, mutations are important for the variation of the general population.

HESI Biology Practice Questions

1. Which molecule is the simplest form of sugar?
    a. Monosaccharide
    b. Fatty acid
    c. Polysaccharide
    d. Amino acid

2. Which type of macromolecule contains genetic information that can be passed to subsequent generations?
    a. Carbohydrates
    b. Lipids
    c. Proteins
    d. Nucleic acids

3. What is the primary unit of inheritance between generations of an organism?
    a. Chromosome
    b. Gene
    c. Gamete
    d. Atom

4. Which one of Mendel's laws theorizes that the alleles for different traits are NOT linked and can be inherited independently of one another?
    a. The Law of Dominance
    b. The Law of Segregation
    c. The Law of Independent Assortment
    d. The Law of Meiosis

5. What does an element's atomic number indicate?
    a. The number of protons
    b. The number of electrons
    c. The number of protons and neutrons
    d. The charge of the element

6. Which of the following is NOT a characteristic of each electron orbital?
    a. The principal quantum number
    b. The angular momentum quantum number
    c. The number of protons inside
    d. The magnetic quantum number

7. Which of the following is a distinct characteristic of a gas?
    a. It has a fixed shape.
    b. It is easy to compress.
    c. It has an exact volume.
    d. The molecules are packed together tightly.

8. Which characteristic of a liquid allows it to have surface tension?
   a. It has adhesion.
   b. It molds to the shape of its container.
   c. It has an exact volume.
   d. It has cohesion.

9. Which type of solid has a symmetrical pattern of molecules within it?
   a. Crystalline
   b. Plastic
   c. Rubber
   d. Amorphous

10. Which characteristic of lipids causes them to not mix with water molecules?
    a. Hydrophobic
    b. Hydrophilic
    c. Insulate the body
    d. Phosphate group

11. Which layer of protein structure is responsible for the sequence of the amino acids?
    a. Secondary
    b. Quaternary
    c. Primary
    d. Tertiary

12. In which type of reaction are complex molecules broken down into smaller, simpler molecules?
    a. Anabolic
    b. Enzymatic
    c. Catabolic
    d. Endergonic

13. Which molecule is an essential part of all metabolic pathways?
    a. Oxygen
    b. Glucose
    c. Protein
    d. ATP

14. What feature do plant cells have that is lacking in animal cells?
    a. Phospholipid bilayer cell membrane
    b. Cell wall
    c. Mitochondria
    d. Golgi apparatus

15. What part of the cell contains the cell's DNA?
    a. Nucleus
    b. Endoplasmic reticulum
    c. Ribosomes
    d. Cell membrane

16. Which molecule starts the citric acid cycle?
    a. ATP
    b. Oxygen
    c. Pyruvate
    d. NADH

17. What is one type of molecule that is used to transport electrons in anaerobic respiration?
    a. Sulfate
    b. Oxygen
    c. Carbon dioxide
    d. ATP

18. Which substance is converted into chemical energy during photosynthesis?
    a. Glucose
    b. Light
    c. Pyruvate
    d. Chlorophyll

19. Which is NOT a phase of the Calvin cycle of photosynthesis?
    a. Carbon fixation
    b. Reduction
    c. Regeneration of the CO_2 acceptor
    d. Light reactions

20. Why is cellular reproduction essential for an organism?
    a. It allows for the replacement of dying and damaged cells.
    b. It marks the end of the organism's life.
    c. It marks the end of growth for an organism.
    d. It makes changes to the organism's DNA.

21. What are the string-like structures that humans carry their genetic information on called?
    a. Genes
    b. Chromosomes
    c. Nuclear envelope
    d. Diploid cell

22. In which situation does codominance of alleles occur?
    a. A third phenotype is generated when two different alleles are present.
    b. There is only one type of allele.
    c. There is one allele with a more prominent phenotype than the other allele.
    d. Both alleles of the gene are expressed equally.

23. Which pairing represents a correct DNA base pairing?
    a. Adenine-guanine
    b. Adenine-cytosine
    c. Guanine-cytosine
    d. Thymine-guanine

24. When is a mutation considered hereditary?
    a. When the sequence was present in the parent gene
    b. When the alteration occurred during the replication process
    c. If it causes a developmental problem
    d. If it is a common occurrence in the population

25. Which carbohydrate consists of 1,700 to 600,000 glucose units, is not soluble in water, and can be stored for long periods of time?
    a. Monomers
    b. Pyruvate
    c. Steroid
    d. Glycogen

For questions 26–30:

There are four stages in cell division: gap 1 (G1), synthesis (S), gap 2 (G2), and mitosis (M). The cell prepares for division in interphase during the G1, S, and G2 phases. Mitosis is when two cells form from the division of one cell.

The graph below shows the percentage of time a typical cell spends in each of these phases:

Cell Phases

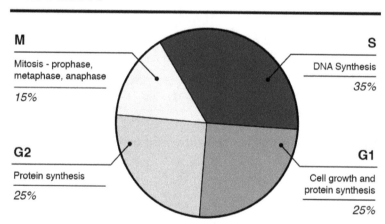

M
Mitosis - prophase, metaphase, anaphase
15%

S
DNA Synthesis
35%

G2
Protein synthesis
25%

G1
Cell growth and protein synthesis
25%

The figure below shows cyclin levels during cell cycle. Cyclins are a class of proteins that control cell division in mammalian cells:

Cell Cycle Stage

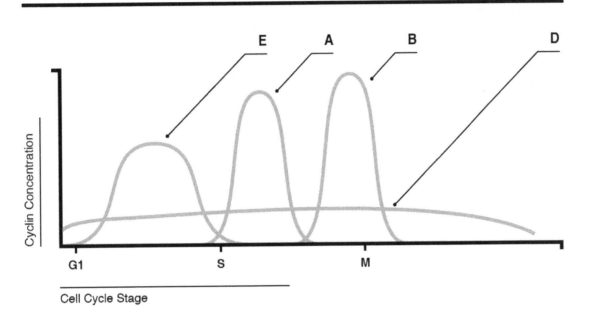

Cell Cycle Stage

26. A fibroblast (a mammalian cell) takes twenty-four hours to divide. How many hours would a fibroblast spend in mitosis?
   a. 12.0
   b. 8.4
   c. 6.0
   d. 3.6

27. Which of the following could be asserted regarding a mammalian cell beginning mitosis?
   a. Cyclin A must be increasing
   b. Cyclin B must be decreasing
   c. Cyclin A must be at its maximum level
   d. Cyclin E must be at its maximum level

28. Which cyclins MOST likely initiate the cell cycle?
   a. Only Cyclin A
   b. Only Cyclin B
   c. Only Cyclin E
   d. Only Cyclin A and Cyclin B

29. Which cyclin seems to have the LEAST effect on any phase of the mammalian cell cycle?
   a. Cyclin A
   b. Cyclin B
   c. Cyclin D
   d. Cyclin E

30. An increase in Cyclin A triggers which of the cell phases?
   a. Protein synthesis
   b. Mitosis
   c. DNA synthesis
   d. Cell growth

Answer Explanations

1. A: Monosaccharides are the simplest sugars that make up carbohydrates. They are important for cellular respiration. Fatty acids, Choice *B*, make up lipids. Polysaccharides, Choice *C*, are larger molecules with repeating monosaccharide units. Amino acids, Choice *D*, are the building blocks of proteins.

2. D: Nucleic acids include DNA and RNA, which are strands of nucleotides that contain genetic information. Carbohydrates, Choice *A*, are made up of sugars that provide energy to the body. Lipids, Choice *B*, are hydrocarbon chains that make up fats. Proteins, Choice *C*, are made up of amino acids that help with many functions for maintaining life.

3. B: Genes are the primary unit of inheritance between generations of an organism. Humans each have twenty-three pairs of chromosomes, Choice *A*, and each chromosome contains hundreds to thousands of genes. Genes each control a specific trait of the organism. Gametes, Choice *C*, are the reproductive cells that contain all of the genetic information of an individual. Atoms, Choice *D*, are the small units that make up all substances.

4. C: The Law of Independent Assortment states that the alleles for different traits are inherited independently of one another. For example, the alleles for eye color are not linked to the alleles for hair color. So, someone could have blue eyes and brown hair or blue eyes and blond hair. The Law of Dominance, Choice *A*, states that one allele has a stronger effect on phenotype than the other allele. The Law of Segregation, Choice *B*, states that each trait has two versions that can be inherited. Each parent contributes one of its alleles, selected randomly, to the daughter offspring. The Law of Meiosis is a fictitious item.

5. A: An element's atomic number refers to the number of protons in the element. The atomic number of each element is unique. The number of protons and neutrons together, Choice *C*, are the nucleons of the element. When an element has a non-neutral charge, it is referred to as an *ion*.

6. C: Electron orbitals only contain electrons. Protons and neutrons reside in the nucleus of an atom. The principal quantum number refers to the size of the orbital. The angular momentum quantum number denotes the shape of the orbital. The magnetic quantum number denotes the orientation of the orbital in space.

7. B: Gases are easy to compress. Their molecules spread out to fill the container they are in, but they can be pushed together so that the space between the molecules decreases. Solids have a fixed shape; therefore, Choice *A* is incorrect. Liquids and solids both have an exact volume, so Choice *C* is not correct. Molecules are generally packed together tightly in solids, which makes Choice *D* incorrect.

8. D: Cohesion is the attraction of liquid molecules to each other. They stick together and create an extra strong bond between them, which allows surface tension to form on top of the liquid. Adhesion, Choice *A*, describes the attraction of a liquid to the container it is in. The shape and volume of the liquid, Choices *B* and *C*, do not affect surface tension.

9. A: Crystalline solids have molecules arranged in a symmetrical pattern. The bonds within the solid are of equal strength, and they break along straight lines. Amorphous solids, Choice *D*, have heterogeneous compositions, so their bonds are not of equal strength, and they do not break evenly. Plastic and rubber, Choices *B* and *C*, are examples of amorphous solids.

10. A: Lipids are made up of long hydrocarbon chains. When mixed with water, the water molecules bind to each other and exclude the lipids. When oil and water are mixed, you can see oil drops floating at the water's surface. Phospholipids have a phosphate group attached to them, which makes that end of the molecule hydrophilic, meaning it associates with water; therefore, Choices *B* and *D* are incorrect. Although lipids do insulate the body, Choice *C*, this characteristic is unrelated to lipids being hydrophobic.

11. C: The primary structure of proteins refers to the sequence of amino acids. The secondary structure, Choice *A*, refers to the folds and coils of the polypeptide backbone. The quaternary structure, Choice *B*, refers to the overall shape the protein has when there is more than one polypeptide chain involved. The tertiary structure, Choice *D*, refers to the shape of the molecule that is generated by the interactions of the side molecules attached to the polypeptide backbone.

12. C: Catabolic reactions entail the breakdown of complex molecules into smaller molecules, with more energy being released at the end of the reaction with the products than was needed to start the reaction. Anabolic reactions, Choice *A*, are those that involve smaller molecules being combined to form larger molecules. Enzymes, Choice *B*, are used in most reactions, anabolic and catabolic. Endergonic reactions require an input of energy, so they are often anabolic, not catabolic. Thus, they are more likely to involve synthesizing larger molecules from smaller constituents.

13. D: ATP is used by most organisms as a direct source of energy. Anaerobic organisms do not use oxygen at all for generating ATP, Choice *A*. The breakdown of glucose, Choice *B*, generates ATP, but it is not involved in all metabolic reactions. Proteins, Choice *C*, can be stored and broken down at later times to produce energy but are also not involved in all metabolic reactions.

14. B: Plant cells are surrounded by a cell wall made up of fibrous polysaccharides and proteins in addition to a phospholipid bilayer membrane, Choice *A*, which is all that animal cells have. Both animal and plant cells have mitochondria and Golgi apparatuses; therefore, Choices *C* and *D* are incorrect.

15. A: A cell's DNA is contained within the nucleus of the cell. The nucleus is surrounded by a protective double membrane called the *nuclear envelope*. The endoplasmic reticulum, Choice *B*, is responsible for synthetic activities of the cell. The ribosomes, Choice *C*, produce proteins. The cell membrane, Choice *D*, surrounds the cell and protects it from the environment.

16. C: Before the citric acid cycle starts, glucose converts to pyruvate, which is the molecule that enters the citric acid cycle. ATP and NADH, Choices *A* and *D*, are both generated by the citric acid cycle. Oxygen molecules, Choice *B*, are used to transport electrons during oxidative phosphorylation.

17. A: Sulfate accepts electrons at the end of the electron transport chain in anaerobic respiration. Nitrate is another molecule that accepts electrons in anaerobic respiration. Anaerobic respiration occurs completely without the use of oxygen, Choice *B*. Carbon dioxide, Choice *C*, is not used during this process. ATP, Choice *D*, is generated at the end of anaerobic respiration.

18. B: Photosynthesis is the process of converting light energy into chemical energy. It occurs in the chloroplasts of plants, which are filled with chlorophyll, Choice *D*. Glucose and pyruvate, Choices *A* and *C*, are often used as an energy source but not during photosynthesis.

19. D: The light reactions occur before the Calvin cycle starts. Carbon fixation, reduction, and regeneration of the CO_2 acceptor, Choices *A*, *B*, and *C*, are all part of the Calvin cycle, which helps convert CO_2 to sucrose, which can be used as a direct energy source for the plant.

20. A: Cellular reproduction is the process of a cell making new cells with similar or the same contents as themselves. As the organism grows, it produces more cells and allows for replacement of cells that have aged or are damaged. It does not mark the end of the organism's life, Choice *B*, or mark the end of growth, as it must grow to reproduce, Choice *C*. Cellular reproduction does not always introduce changes to an organism's DNA; this occurs only if mutations occur. Therefore, Choice *D* is incorrect.

21. B: Chromosomes are the string-like structures that contain all of a human's genetic information. Each human has twenty-three chromosomes, and each chromosome contains between a few hundred and a few thousand genes. Genes, Choice *A*, each encode a specific trait. Chromosomes are contained within the nucleus of the cell, which is surrounded by a nuclear envelope, which makes Choice *C* incorrect. Diploid cells contain forty-six chromosomes during reproduction; therefore, Choice *D* is incorrect.

22. D: In codominance, both alleles of a gene are expressed equally. A cow that has one red hair allele and one white hair allele has a coat that is red and white, not pink. In incomplete dominance, the presence of one white hair allele and one red hair allele would create pink hair, Choice *A*. Generally, in genetics, there is one dominant allele and one recessive allele, Choice *C*. All genes have two allele choices, so Choice *B* does not occur in normal genetics.

23. C: Guanine and cytosine pair together in DNA, as do adenine and thymine. The pairings are based on the hydrogen bonds that can form between the bases. They fit together well and can form tight helices based on their configurations.

24. A: Hereditary mutations are passed down from the parent gene, where the sequence alteration was already present. Choice *B* refers to acquired mutations, which occur when the sequence alteration happens during the replication process. Some mutations can cause developmental problems, but they are not linked to being hereditary or not; therefore, Choice *C* is incorrect. Mutations do not occur commonly in the population, which makes Choice *D* incorrect.

25. D: Glycogen is a long polymer of glucose molecules. It can be broken down into individual glucose molecules to provide energy to the body. Monomers, Choice *A*, are the smallest of sugar molecules. Pyruvate, Choice *B*, is the carbohydrate that starts the citric acid cycle. Steroids, Choice *C*, are a type of lipid.

26. D: Looking at Figure 1 shows that mitosis takes up 15 percent of the entire cycle, and 15 percent of twenty-four hours is 3.6 hours.

27. B: Looking at Figure 2 shows that Cyclin B is decreasing during the mitosis (M) stage of the cell cycle.

28. C: Looking at Figure 2, Cyclin E is the only choice that is present at the beginning of the cell cycle.

29. C: Looking at Figure 2, Cyclin D is the only choice that seems to be steady throughout the entire cell cycle; thus, Cyclin D will most likely have the least effect on the cycle.

30. C: Looking at Figure 2, the increase in Cyclin A happens at the S phase of the cell cycle. Referencing the cycle components in Figure 1 shows that DNA synthesis is the only occurrence in Phase S.

Chemistry

Scientific Notation, the Metric System, and Temperature Scales

Scientific Notation

Scientific notation is a system used to represent numbers that are very large or very small. Sometimes, numbers are way too big or small to be written out with multiple zeros behind them or in decimal form, so scientific notation is used as a way to express these numbers in a simpler way.

Scientific notation takes the decimal notation and turns it into scientific notation, like the table below:

Decimal Notation	Scientific Notation
5	5×10^0
500	5×10^2
10,000,000	1×10^7
8,000,000,000	8×10^9
-55,000	-5.5×10^4
.00001	10^{-5}

In scientific notation, the decimal is placed after the first digit and all the remaining numbers are dropped. For example, 5 becomes "5.0×10^0." This equation is raised to the zero power because there are no zeros behind the number "5." Always put the decimal after the first number. Let's say we have the number 125,000. We would write this using scientific notation as follows: 1.25×10^5, because to move the decimal from behind "1" to behind "125,000" takes five counts, so we put the exponent "5" behind the "10." As you can see in the table above, the number ".00001" is too cumbersome to be written out each time for an equation, so we would want to say that it is "10^{-5}." If we count from the place behind the decimal point to the number "1," we see that we go backwards 5 places. Thus, the "-5" in the scientific notation form represents 5 places to the right of the decimal.

Converting Within the Metric System

Recall that the metric system has base units of meter for length, kilogram for mass, and liter for liquid volume. This system expands to three places above the base unit and three places below. These places correspond with prefixes with a base of 10. The following table shows the conversions:

kilo-	hecto-	deka-	base	deci-	centi-	milli-
1,000 times the base	100 times the base	10 times the base		1/10 times the base	1/100 times the base	1/1000 times the base

Temperature Scales

Science utilizes three primary temperature scales. The temperature scale most often used in the United States is the Fahrenheit (F) scale. The Fahrenheit scale uses key markers based on the measurements of the freezing (32 °F) and boiling (212 °F) points of water. In the United States, when taking a person's temperature with a thermometer, the Fahrenheit scale is used to represent this information. The human body registers an average temperature of 98.6 °F.

Another temperature scale commonly used in science is the Celsius (C) scale (also called *centigrade* because the overall scale is divided into one hundred parts). The Celsius scale marks the temperature for water freezing at 0 °C and boiling at 100 °C. The average temperature of the human body registers at 37 °C. Most countries in the world use the Celsius scale for everyday temperature measurements.

For scientists to easily communicate information regarding temperature, an overall standard temperature scale was agreed upon. This scale is the Kelvin (K) scale. Named for Lord Kelvin, who conducted research in thermodynamics, the Kelvin scale contains the largest range of temperatures to facilitate any possible readings.

The **Kelvin scale** is the accepted measurement by the International System of Units (from the French *Système international d'unités*), or SI, for temperature. The Kelvin scale is employed in thermodynamics, and its reading for 0 is the basis for absolute zero. This scale is rarely used for measuring temperatures in the medical field.

The conversions between the temperature scales are as follows:

Degrees Fahrenheit to Degrees Celsius:

$$^0C = \frac{5}{9}(^0F - 32)$$

Degrees Celsius to Degrees Fahrenheit:

$$^0F = \frac{9}{5}(^\circ C) + 32$$

Degrees Celsius to Kelvin:

$$K = \,^0C + 273.15$$

For example, if a patient has a temperature of 38 °C, what would this be on the Fahrenheit scale?

Solution:

First, select the correct conversion equation from the list above.

$$^0F = \frac{9}{5}(^\circ C) + 32$$

Next, plug in the known value for °C, 38.

$$^0F = \frac{9}{5}(38) + 32$$

Finally, calculate the desired value for °F.

$$^0F = \frac{9}{5}(38) + 32$$

$$°F = 100.4°F$$

For example, what would the temperature 52 °C be on the Kelvin scale?

First, select the correct conversion equation from the list above.

$$K = {}^{0}C + 273.15$$

Next, plug in the known value for °C, 52.

$$K = 52 + 273.15$$

Finally, calculate the desired value for K.

$$K = 325.15\ K$$

Atomic Structure and the Periodic Table

Today's primary model of the atom was proposed by scientist Niels Bohr. **Bohr's atomic model** consists of a nucleus, or core, which is made up of positively charged protons and neutrally charged neutrons. Neutrons are theorized to be in the nucleus with the protons to provide "balance" and stability to the protons at the center of the atom. More than 99 percent of the mass of an atom is found in the nucleus. Orbitals surrounding the nucleus contain negatively charged particles called *electrons*. Since the entire structure of an atom is too small to be seen with the unaided eye, an electron microscope is required for detection. Even with such magnification, the actual particles of the atom are not visible.

An atom has an atomic number that is determined by the number of protons within the nucleus. Some substances are made up of atoms, all with the same atomic number. Such a substance is called an *element*. Using their atomic numbers, elements are organized and grouped by similar properties in a chart called the *Periodic Table*.

If the total number of protons is added to the total number of neutrons in an atom, this sum provides the atom's mass number. Most atoms have a nucleus that is electronically neutral, and all atoms of one type have the same atomic number. There are some atoms of the same type that have a different mass number. The variation in the mass number is due to an imbalance of neutrons within the nucleus of the atoms. If atoms have this variance in neutrons, they are called *isotopes*. It is the different number of neutrons that gives such atoms a different mass number.

A concise method of arranging elements by atomic number, similar characteristics, and electron configurations in a tabular format was necessary to represent elements. This was originally organized by scientist Dmitri Mendeleev using the Periodic Table. The vertical lines on the Periodic Table are called *columns* and are sorted by similar chemical properties/characteristics, such as appearance and reactivity. This is observed in the shiny texture of metals, the softness of post-transition metals, and the high melting points of alkali earth metals. The horizontal lines on the Periodic Table are called *rows* and are arranged by electron valance configurations. The columns are referred to as *groups*, and the rows are *periods*.

Elements are set by ascending atomic number, from left to right. The number of protons contained within the nucleus of the atom is represented by the atomic number. For example, hydrogen has one proton in its nucleus, so it has an atomic number of 1.

The Periodic Table of the Elements

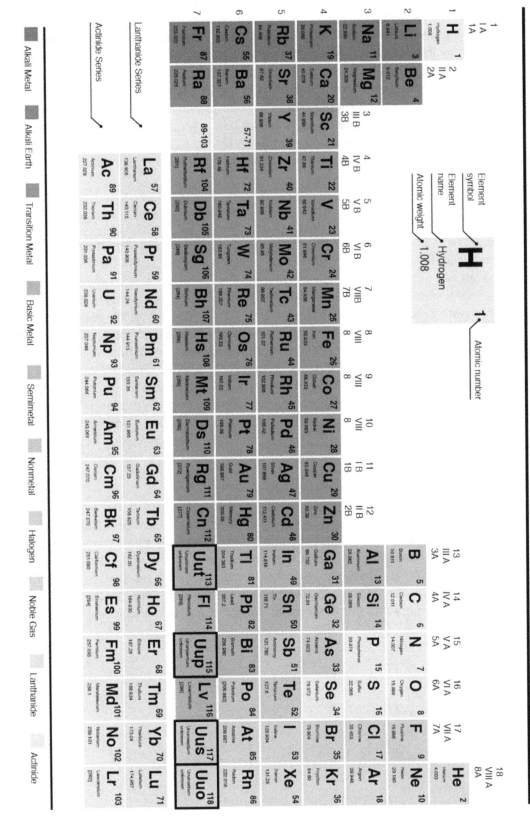

Since isotopes can have different masses within the same type of element, the atomic mass of an element is the average mass of all the naturally occurring atoms of that given element. Atomic mass is calculated by finding the relative abundance of isotopes that might be used in chemistry. A different number referred to as the mass number is found by adding the number of protons and neutrons of an atom together. For example, the mass number of one typical chlorine atom is 35: the nucleus has 17 protons (given by chlorine's atomic number of 17) and 18 neutrons. However, a large number of chlorine isotopes with a mass number of 37 exist in nature. These isotopes have 20 neutrons instead of 18 neutrons. The average of all the mass numbers turns out to be 35.5 amu, which is chlorine's atomic mass on the periodic table. In contrast, a typical carbon atom has a mass number of 12, and its atomic mass is 12.01 amu because there are not as many naturally occurring isotopes that raise the average number, as observed with chlorine.

Chemical Equations

Chemical equations describe how the molecules are changed when the chemical reaction occurs. For example, the chemical equation of the hexane combustion reaction is $2C_6H_{14} + 17O_2 \rightarrow 12CO_2 + 14H_2O$. The "+" sign on the left side of the equation indicates that those molecules are reacting with each other, and the arrow, "$\rightarrow$," in the middle of the equation indicates that the reactants are producing something else. The coefficient before a molecule indicates the quantity of that specific molecule that is present for the reaction. The subscript next to an element indicates the quantity of that element in each molecule. In order for the chemical equation to be balanced, the quantity of each element on both sides of the equation should be equal. For example, in the hexane equation above, there are twelve carbon elements, twenty-eight hydrogen elements, and thirty-four oxygen elements on each side of the equation. Even though they are part of different molecules on each side, the overall quantity is the same. The state of matter of the reactants and products can also be included in a chemical equation and would be written in parentheses next to each element as follows: gas (g), liquid (l), solid (s), and dissolved in water, or aqueous (aq).

Reaction Rates, Equilibrium, and Reversibility

The rate of a chemical reaction can be increased by adding a catalyst to the reaction. Catalysts are substances that lower the activation energy required to go from the reactants to the products of the reaction but are not consumed in the process. The activation energy of a reaction is the minimum amount of energy that is required to make the reaction move forward and change the reactants into the products. When catalysts are present, less energy is required to complete the reaction. For example, hydrogen peroxide will eventually decompose into two water molecules and one oxygen molecule.

If potassium permanganate is added to the reaction, the decomposition happens at a much faster rate. Similarly, increasing the temperature or pressure in the environment of the reaction can increase the rate of the reaction. Higher temperatures increase the number of high-energy collisions that lead to the products. The same happens when increasing pressure for gaseous reactants, but not with solid or liquid reactants. Increasing the concentration of the reactants or the available surface area over which they can react also increases the rate of the reaction.

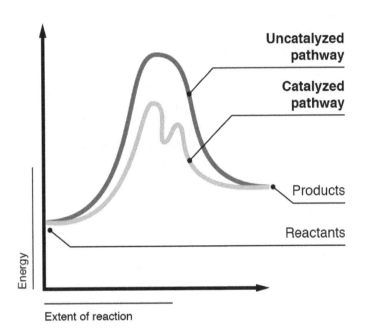

Many reactions are *reversible,* which means that the products can revert back to the reactants under certain conditions. In such reactions, the arrow will be double-headed, indicating that the reaction can proceed in either direction. Reactions reach a state of *equilibrium* when the net concentration of the reactants and products are not changing. This does not mean that the reactions have stopped occurring, but that there is no overall change in either direction (forming more product from the reactants or the product undergoing the reverse reaction to re-form the reactants). Some number of reactions may be going on in both directions, but they cancel each other out so that there is no net change in concentrations on either side of the reaction arrow.

Solutions and Solubility

A *solution* is a homogenous mixture of two or more substances. Unlike heterogenous mixtures, in solutions, the *solute,* which is a substance that can be dissolved, is uniformly distributed throughout the *solvent,* which is the substance in which the solvent dissolves. For example, when 10 grams of table salt (NaCl) is added to a 100 mL of room temperature water and then stirred until all of the salt (the solute) has dissolved in the water (the solvent), a solution is formed. The dissolved salt, in the form of Na^+ and Cl^- ions, will be evenly distributed throughout the water. In this case, the solution is *diluted* because only a small amount of solute was dissolved in a comparatively large volume of solvent. The salt water solution would be said to be *concentrated* if a large amount of salt was added, stirred, and dissolved into the water, 30 grams, for example. When more solute is added to the solvent but even after stirring, some settles on the bottom without dissolving, the solution is *saturated.* For example, in 100 mL of room temperature water, about 35 grams of table salt can dissolve before the solution is saturated. Beyond this point—called the saturation point—any additional salt added will not readily dissolve. Sometimes, it is possible to temporarily dissolve excessive solute in the solvent, which creates a *supersaturated* solution. However, as soon as this solution is disturbed, the process of *crystallization* will begin and a solid will begin precipitating out of the solution.

It is often necessary, for example when working with chemicals or mixing acids and bases, to quantitatively determine the concentration of a solution, which is a more precise measure than using qualitative terms like *diluted*, *concentrated*, *saturated*, and *supersaturated*. The *molarity, c,* of a solution is a measure of its concentration; specifically, it is the number of moles of solute (represented by *n* in the formula) per liter of solution *(V)*. Therefore, the following is the formula for calculating the molarity of a solution:

$$c = \frac{n}{V}$$

It is important to remember that the volume in the denominator of the equation above is in liters of solution, not solvent. Adding solute increases the volume of the entire solution, so the molarity formula accounts for this volumetric increase.

Factors Affecting Solubility

Solubility refers to a solvent's ability to dissolve a solute. Certain factors can affect solubility, such as temperature and pressure. Depending on the state of matter of the molecules in the solution, these factors may increase or decrease solubility. When most people think of solutions, they imagine a solid or liquid solute dissolved in a liquid solvent, like water. However, solutions can be composed on molecules in the other states of matter as well. The following are examples of solutions involving combinations of solids, liquids, and gasses:

- Dry air is solution of gasses, mainly nitrogen and oxygen, with carbon dioxide and others as well

- Vinegar is a solution of liquid acetic acid and liquid water

- Brass is a solution of solid copper and solid zinc

- Amalgams can be a solution of liquid mercury with a solid metal like gold

- Hummingbirds like sweet water, a solution of liquid water and solid sucrose (table sugar)

Increases in temperature, tend to increase a solute's solubility, except in the case of gasses wherein higher temperature reduce the solubility of gaseous solutions and gasses dissolved in water. However, the solubility of gasses in organic solvents increases with increases in temperature. Pressure is directly related to the solubility of gasses, but not of liquids or solids. Agitating, or stirring, a solution does not affect solubility, but it does increase the rate at which the solute dissolves.

The *electronegativities*, or *polarities,* of the solvent and solute determine whether the solute will readily dissolve in the solvent. The key to the potential for a solution to form and the solute to dissolve in the solvent is "like dissolves like." If the solute is polar, it will dissolve in a polar solvent. If the solute is non-polar, it will dissolve in a non-polar solvent. Water is an example of a polar solvent, while benzene is an example of a non-polar solvent.

Chemical Reactions

A **chemical reaction** is a process that involves a change in the molecular arrangement of a substance. Generally, one set of chemical substances, called the reactants, is rearranged into a different set of chemical substances, called the products, by the breaking and re-forming of bonds between atoms. In a chemical reaction, it is important to realize that no new atoms or molecules are introduced. The products are formed solely from the atoms and molecules that are present in the reactants. These can involve a change in state of matter as well. Making glass, burning fuel, and brewing beer are all examples of chemical reactions.

Generally, chemical reactions are thought to involve changes in positions of electrons with the breaking and re-forming of chemical bonds, without changes to the nucleus of the atoms. The three main types of chemical reactions are combination, decomposition, and combustion.

Combination

In **combination reactions**, two or more reactants are combined to form one more complex, larger product. The bonds of the reactants are broken, the elements are arranged, and then new bonds are formed between all of the elements to form the product. It can be written as A + B → C, where A and B are the reactants and C is the product. An example of a combination reaction is the creation of iron(II) sulfide from iron and sulfur, which is written as:

$$8Fe + S8 \rightarrow 8FeS$$

Decomposition

Decomposition reactions are almost the opposite of combination reactions. They occur when one substance is broken down into two or more products. The bonds of the first substance are broken, the elements are rearranged, and then the elements are bonded together in new configurations to make two or more molecules. These reactions can be written as C → B + A, where C is the reactant and A and B are the products. An example of a decomposition reaction is the electrolysis of water to make oxygen and hydrogen gas, which is written as:

$$2H2O \rightarrow 2H2 + O2$$

Combustion

Combustion reactions are a specific type of chemical reaction that involves oxygen gas as a reactant. This mostly involves the burning of a substance. The combustion of hexane in air is one example of a combustion reaction. The hexane gas combines with oxygen in the air to form carbon dioxide and water. The reaction can be written as:

$$2C6H14 + 17O2 \rightarrow 12CO2 + 14H2O$$

Stoichiometry

Stoichiometry uses proportions based on the principles of the conservation of mass and the conservation of energy. It deals with first balancing the chemical (and sometimes physical) changes in a reaction and then finding the ratios of the reactants used and what products resulted. Just as there are different types of reactions, there are different types of stoichiometry problems. Different reactions can involve mass, volume, or moles in varying combinations. The steps to solve a stoichiometry problem are to first, balance the equation; next, find the number of total products; and finally, calculate the desired information regarding molar mass, percent yield, etc.

The molar mass of any substance is the measure of the mass of one mole of that substance. For pure elements, the molar mass is also referred to as the *atomic mass unit (amu)* for that substance. In compounds, this is calculated by adding the molar mas of each substance in the compound. For example, the molar mass of carbon can be found on the Periodic Table as 12.01 g/mol, while finding the molar mass of water (H_2O) requires a bit of calculation.

$$
\begin{aligned}
\text{the molar mass of hydrogen} &= 1.01 \times 2 = 2.02 \\
+ \text{ the molar mass of oxygen} &= 16.0 \quad\quad = +16.00 \\
&\hspace{3cm} \overline{18.02 \text{ g/mol}}
\end{aligned}
$$

To determine the percent composition of a compound, the individual molar masses of each component need to be divided by the total molar mass of the compound and then multiplied by 100. For example, to find the percent composition of carbon dioxide (CO_2) first requires the calculation of the molar mass of CO_2.

$$
\begin{aligned}
\text{the molar mass of carbon} &= 12.01 \quad\quad = 12.01 \\
+ \text{ the molar mass of oxygen} &= 16.0 \times 2 = +32.00 \\
&\hspace{3cm} \overline{44.01 \text{ g/mol}}
\end{aligned}
$$

Next, take each individual mass, divide by the total mass of the compound, and then multiply by 100 to get the percent composition of each component.

$$
\frac{12.01 \ g/mol}{44.01 \ g/mol} = 0.2729 \times 100 = 27.29\% \ carbon
$$

$$
\frac{32.00 \ g/mol}{44.01 \ g/mol} = 0.7271 \times 100 = 72.71\% \ oxygen
$$

A quick check in the addition of the percentages should always total 100%.

If an example provides the basis for an equation, the equation would first need to be balanced to calculate any proportions. For example, if 15 g of C_2H_6 reacts with 64 g of O_2, how many grams of CO_2 will be formed?

First, write the chemical equation:

$$C_2H_6 + O_2 \rightarrow CO_2 + H_2O$$

Next, balance the equation:

$$2\,C_2H_6 + 7\,O_2 \rightarrow 4\,CO_2 + 6\,H_2O$$

Then, calculate the desired amount based on the beginning information of 15 g of C_2H_6:

$$15 \ g \ C_2H_6 \times \frac{1 \ mole \ C_2H_6}{30 \ g \ C_2H_6} \times \frac{4 \ moles \ CO_2}{2 \ moles \ C_2H_6} \times \frac{44 \ g \ CO_2}{1 \ mole \ CO_2} = 44 \ g \ CO_2$$

To check that this would be the smaller amount (or how much until one of the reactants is used up, thus ending the reaction), the calculation would need to be done for the 64 g of O_2:

$$64 \; g \; O_2 \times \frac{1 \; mole \; O_2}{32 \; g \; O_2} \times \frac{4 \; moles \; CO_2}{7 \; moles \; O_2} \times \frac{44 \; g \; CO_2}{1 \; mole \; CO_2} = 50.5 \; g \; CO_2$$

The yield from the C_2H_6 is smaller, so it would be used up first, ending the reaction. This calculation would determine the maximum amount of CO_2 that could possibly be produced.

Oxidation and Reduction

Oxidation/reduction (redox or half) reactions involve the oxidation of one species and the reduction of the other species in the reactants of a chemical equation. This can be seen through three main types of transfers.

The first type is through the transfer of oxygen. The reactant gaining an oxygen is the oxidizing agent, and the reactant losing an oxygen is the reduction agent.

For example, the oxidation of magnesium is as follows:

$$2 \; Mg(s) + O_2(g) \; \rightarrow \; 2 \; MgO(s)$$

The second type is through the transfer of hydrogen. The reactant losing the hydrogen is the oxidizing agent, and the other reactant is the reduction agent.

For example, the redox of ammonia and bromine results in nitrogen and hydrogen bromide due to bromine gaining a hydrogen as follows:

$$2 \; NH_3 + 3 \; Br_2 \rightarrow \; N_2 + 6 \; HBr$$

The third type is through the loss of electrons from one species, known as the *oxidation agent*, and the gain of electrons to the other species, known as the *reduction agent*. For a reactant to become "oxidized," it must give up an electron.

For example, the redox of copper and silver is as follows:

$$Cu(s) + 2 \; Ag^+(aq) \; \rightarrow \; Cu^{2+}(aq) + 2 \; Ag(s)$$

It is also important to note that the oxidation numbers can change in a redox reaction due to the transfer of oxygen atoms. Standard rules for finding the oxidation numbers for a compound are listed below:

1. The oxidation number of a free element is always 0.

2. The oxidation number of a monatomic ion equals the charge of the ion.

3. The oxidation number of H is +1, but it is –1 when combined with less electronegative elements.

4. The oxidation number of O in compounds is usually –2, but it is –1 in peroxides.

5. The oxidation number of a Group 1 element in a compound is +1.

6. The oxidation number of a Group 2 element in a compound is +2.

7. The oxidation number of a Group 17 element in a binary compound is –1.

8. The sum of the oxidation numbers of all the atoms in a neutral compound is 0.

9. The sum of the oxidation numbers in a polyatomic ion is equal to the charge of the ion.

These rules can be applied to determine the oxidation number of an unknown component of a compound.

For example, what is the oxidation number of Cr in $CrCl_3$?

From rule 7, the oxidation number of Cl is given as –1. Since there are 3 chlorines in this compound, that would equal 3×-1 for a result of –3. According to rule 8, the total oxidation number of Cr must balance the total oxidation number of Cl, so Cr must have a total oxidation number equaling +3 ($-3 + +3 = 0$). There is only 1 Cr, so the oxidation number would be multiplied by 1, or the same as the total of +3, written as follows:

$$\overset{+3 \quad -1}{\underset{+3 \quad -3}{CrCl_3}}$$

Acids and Bases

If something has a sour taste, it is considered acidic, and if something has a bitter taste, it is considered basic. Acids and bases are generally identified by the reaction they have when combined with water. An acid will increase the concentration of hydrogen ions (H^+) in water, and a base will increase the concentration of hydroxide ions (OH^-). Other methods of identification with various indicators have been designed over the years.

To better categorize the varying strength levels of acids and bases, the pH scale is employed. The pH scale is a logarithmic (base 10) grading applied to acids and bases according to their strength. The pH scale contains values from 0 through 14 and uses 7 as neutral. If a solution registers below a 7 on the pH scale, it is considered an acid. If a solution registers higher than a 7, it is considered a base. To perform a quick test on a solution, litmus paper can be used. A base will turn red litmus paper blue, and an acid will turn blue litmus paper red. To gauge the strength of an acid or base, a test using phenolphthalein can be administered. An acid will turn red phenolphthalein to colorless, and a base will turn colorless phenolphthalein to pink. As demonstrated with these types of tests, acids and bases neutralize each other. When acids and bases react with one another, they produce salts (also called *ionic substances*).

Acids and bases have varying strengths. For example, if an acid completely dissolves in water and ionizes, forming an H^+ and an anion, it is considered a strong acid. There are only a few common strong acids, including sulfuric (H_2SO_4), hydrochloric (HCl), nitric (HNO_3), hydrobromic (HBr), hydroiodic (HI), and perchloric ($HClO_4$). Other types of acids are considered weak.

An easy way to tell if something is an acid is by looking for the leading "H" in the chemical formula.

A base is considered strong if it completely dissociates into the cation of OH^-, including sodium hydroxide (NaOH), potassium hydroxide (KOH), lithium hydroxide (LiOH), cesium hydroxide (CsOH), rubidium hydroxide (RbOH), barium hydroxide ($Ba(OH)_2$), calcium hydroxide ($Ca(OH)_2$), and strontium hydroxide

$(Sr(OH)_2)$. Just as with acids, other types of bases are considered weak. An easy way to tell if something is a base is by looking for the "OH" ending on the chemical formula.

In pure water, autoionization occurs when a water molecule (H_2O) loses the nucleus of one of the two hydrogen atoms to become a hydroxide ion (OH^-). The nucleus then pairs with another water molecule to form hydronium (H_3O^+). This autoionization process shows that water is *amphoteric*, which means it can react as an acid or as a base.

Pure water is considered neutral, but the presence of any impurities can throw off this neutral balance, causing the water to be slightly acidic or basic. This can include the exposure of water to air, which can introduce carbon dioxide molecules to form carbonic acid (H_2CO_3), thus making the water slightly acidic. Any variation from the middle of the pH scale (7) indicates a non-neutral substance.

Nuclear Chemistry

Nuclear chemistry (also referred to as *nuclear physics*) deals with interactions within the nuclei of atoms. This differs from typical chemical reactions, which involve interactions with the electrons of atoms. If the nucleus of an atom is unstable, it emits radiation as it releases energy resulting from changes in the nucleus. This instability often occurs in isotopes of an element. An isotope is formed when the nucleus of an atom has the same number of protons but a different number of neutrons. This difference in mass causes a heavy, unstable condition in the nucleus.

According to quantum theory, there is no way to precisely predict when an atom will decay, but the decay of a collection of atoms in a substance can be predicted by their collective half-life. Half-life is used to calculate the time it takes for have nuclei in atoms of a radioactive substance to have undergone radioactive decay (in which they emit particles and energy).

There are three primary types of nuclear decay occurring in an atom with an unstable nucleus: alpha, beta, and gamma.

In **alpha decay**, an atom will emit two protons and two neutrons from its nucleus. This emission is in the form of a "bundle" and is called an *alpha particle*. Occurring mainly in larger, heavier atoms, alpha decay causes the atom's proton count to drop by two, thus resulting in the creation of a new element. Alpha radiation is extremely weak and can be blocked by something as thin as a piece of paper.

When the neutron of an atom emits an electron and causes the electron count to increase, the proton count of the nucleus is also increased. This action creates a new element and emits *beta radiation* in the process. Beta radiation is slightly more dangerous than alpha radiation, but it can be blocked by heavy materials such as aluminum or even wood.

The most dangerous type of radiation results from gamma decay. *Gamma decay* does not alter the mass or the charge of an atom. Gamma radiation is emitted along with an alpha or beta particle. It is extremely dangerous and can only be blocked by lead.

For example, iodine is a stable element, often used in nuclear medicine. Iodine's atomic number is 53, and its atomic mass is 127 amu. When an isotope of iodine, with atomic number 53 and atomic mass of 131 amu (due to an excess of four neutrons), is used in the human body, it can be seen in the thyroid as a radioactive tracer.

When naturally-occurring radioactive elements decay, they follow a radioactive decay series, which starts as one element that decays into a second element, which then decays into a third element, and so on until a stable element is finally reached. There are three naturally-occurring radioactive decay series. Each of these series begins with either uranium-235, uranium-238, or thorium. For example, uranium-238 decays into astatine, bismuth, lead, polonium, protactinium, radium, radon, thallium, and thorium before finally becoming a more stable element. An artificial radioactive series begins with the artificially-made element of neptunium and decays into elements such as polonium and americium on its way to becoming more stable.

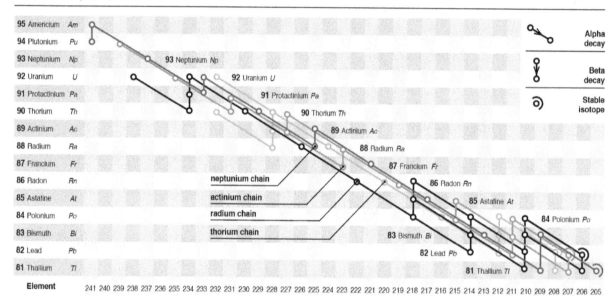

Isotopes can be created through separation and synthesis. There are approximately two hundred radioisotopes; most of them are artificially created. Bombarding the nucleus with nuclear particles or nuclei changes the nucleus of an element. This method is called *transmutation* and has resulted in the formation of new, artificial elements.

The application of half-life knowledge can be seen through the carbon cycle used in carbon dating. Some elements have been estimated to be as old as our universe, and studying the position of something such as carbon in its half-life decay cycle can provide an accurate age of a substance containing carbon. Carbon-14 is utilized for this specific purpose.

The understanding of nuclear chemistry is important for scientists to design and utilize radioactive drugs for treatments and diagnostic techniques. If an isotope is radioactive, it can easily be detected as a contrast agent in the human body, enabling medical professionals to view and diagnose issues that could not be observed without contrast or through physical exams or x-rays. When radioactive tracers are introduced, they can aid in the detection of how systems work. Since the amount of radiation used is small, it can help create a map of its path through a system without causing any disruption to that system.

The radioactive materials can also provide the necessary backdrop or contrast for reading emissions from samples by spectroscopes.

Exposure to radiation has varying effects on the human body. Medical treatments can utilize short exposures to radiation, and damage can be localized to specific, targeted areas, as in treatments for cancer. Extended exposure can cause chromosome damage through breaking the chemical bonds of DNA. Prolonged exposure to radiation can even cause cancer by the mutation and killing of cells and through diminishing the body's ability to produce cells and heal. Overexposure to radiation can result in death.

Biochemistry

The study of the chemistry of living things is called *biochemistry*. Specifically, biochemistry focuses on the molecules and compounds that make up organisms. Analyzing the multiple cycles that organisms undergo for survival is a primary part of biochemistry.

Biochemistry studies cycles such as the following:

- Photosynthesis: Plants use water and carbon dioxide to create simple sugars and oxygen. For example, in the Calvin cycle, structures in chloroplasts are involved in the fixation of carbon dioxide to produce a 6-carbon sugar. Due to its instability, it quickly hydrolyzes to two separate molecules of 3-phosphogylcerate.

- Cellular respiration: Organisms break down sugars, proteins, and starches to create energy and carbon dioxide via glycolysis, the Krebs cycle, the electron transport chain, beta oxidation, etc. For example, in the Krebs cycle, mitochondria take pyruvate molecules (CH_3-CO-COO^-) and, after a series of reaction, produce energy (in the form of ATP) and carbon dioxide.

These cycles involve the production and breakdown of key components in biochemistry, described below.

Carbohydrates are known as *sugars* (COH^-). They are long chains plants create for food storage and structure. Carbohydrates can be seen in the production of shells (containing chitin) and stems (containing cellulose). Sugar is broken down in the mitochondria of a cell to power the creation of adenosine triphosphate (ATP), which is necessary for cell metabolism. Molecules of sugar are called *saccharides* and named in accordance to the number of molecules present. One molecule is called a *monosaccharide*, two molecules together is called a *disaccharide*, three molecules together is called a *trisaccharide*, and so forth. Simple sugars created through photosynthesis are called *glucose* ($C_6H_{12}O_6$). A starch is formed when several carbohydrates combine. The structural basis for most plants is a starch called *cellulose*.

Lipids are a category of molecules that do not mix well with water. This category of lipids contains fats, waxes, and cutin (plant wax that deters evaporation). Triglycerides are formed from three fatty acids, which are carbons connected in long chains, connected to a glycerol backbone. The type of bonds formed in the fatty acid structure of a triglyceride determines the properties of the fat. Saturated fats have only single bond bonds between carbons and are weaker than unsaturated fats, which have at least one double. Saturated fats tend to be solid at room temperature because the single bonds allow all the chains in the structure to pack in more tightly. Unsaturated fats cannot pack together as tightly because kinks are formed in the chain where there are double bonds. This looser arrangement of fatty acid chains causes most unsaturated fats to be liquid at room temperature.

Another category of lipids, called *steroids*, consists of a four-ring structure containing one ring of five carbons and three rings of six carbons. Steroids have very specific molecular structures, which determine their category. Cholesterol is one of the most important biological steroids, which among its many functions, is an integral constituent of cell membranes. Other steroids help form sex hormones or act as anti-inflammatories. Humans can increase their muscle and bone synthesis through anabolic steroids.

Another important area of study in biochemistry is acids. The main type, nucleic acids, are contained within the nucleus of a cell. Nucleic acids contain all the information necessary for cell replication. Specific types of nucleic acid are deoxyribonucleic acid (DNA), ribonucleic acid (RNA), messenger ribonucleic acid (mRNA), transfer ribonucleic acid (tRNA) and ribosomal ribonucleic acid (rRNA). These acids also assist in the building of proteins. DNA is a very complex and long chain composed of two nucleotide strands twisted around each other in a curved ladder configuration (double helix). DNA is the primary component of chromosomes and contains an encoded record of genetic material. This material is transferred along by RNA. DNA is more stable than RNA due to its reduction in more reactive oxygen atoms.

DNA can be broken down into building blocks (monomers), including adenine, thymine, cytosine, and guanine. Uracil is a building block contained only within RNA. All these parts are made of the following three primary components:

- Five carbon sugar; the structure of DNA is missing a hydroxyl group (OH) when compared to the structure of RNA.

- A nitrogen base; there are four, which are grouped into pyrimidines (thymine and cytosine) and purines (guanine and adenine) based on their structures.

- A phosphate ion (PO_4^{3-}), which gives DNA a negative charge.

Amino acids are long molecules made from shorter building blocks. More than five hundred amino acids have been identified, but only twenty of these appear in the genetic code. Amino acids contain a carboxyl group and are used in cells to build proteins. The carboxyl group has a carbon double-bonded to oxygen (COO^-) and a single-bonded hydroxyl (OH) group.

Amino acids (which contain the amine group, NH_2) are categorized as nonessential, conditional, or essential. The human body can synthesize nonessential amino acids such as asparagine, aspartate, and alanine. However, if the human body is stressed or unbalanced from an illness, it may not be able to produce the conditional amino acids. Conditional amino acids include glutamine, arginine, cysteine, glycine, proline, tyrosine, ornithine, and serine. The remaining amino acids must be obtained through diet and are referred to as *essential amino acids*. These include isoleucine, leucine, valine, lysine, phenylalanine, methionine, threonine, and tryptophan. The human body cannot store amino acids, so a daily allowance must be taken/consumed for proper health and function. Many proteins derived from animal sources contain a full complement of the essential amino acids. Some vegetarian options, such as soy (tofu) and quinoa, can also supply the full gamut of essential amino acids, especially when paired together (for example, rice and beans).

Enzymes are catalysts that aid in the breakdown of proteins. Enzymes are necessary for most cellular metabolic processes to occur at rates fast enough to sustain life. There are specific enzymes for every individual task. Enzymes are regulated by temperature, activators, pH levels, and inhibitors.

HESI Chemistry Practice Questions

1. Which of the following is an example of a physical property of substances?
   a. Odor
   b. Reactivity
   c. Flammability
   d. Toxicity

2. Which type of matter has molecules that cannot move within the substance and breaks evenly across a plane due to the symmetry of its molecular arrangement?
   a. Gas
   b. Crystalline solid
   c. Liquid
   d. Amorphous solid

3. What type of reactions involve the breaking and re-forming of bonds between atoms?
   a. Chemical
   b. Physical
   c. Isotonic
   d. Electron

4. When is it helpful to use scientific notation to represent numbers?
   a. When the number is very large or very small
   b. When the number is a multiple of ten
   c. When the number involved in a scientific experiment
   d. For numbers between 0 and 100 only

5. Which of the following units is 10-fold greater than a centimeter?
   a. Millimeter
   b. Foot
   c. Decimeter
   d. Kilometer

6. At what temperature does water boil?
   a. 0 °C
   b. 32 °F
   c. 98.6 °F
   d. 100 °C

7. In which part of the atom is 99 percent of its mass found?
   a. Orbitals
   b. Nucleus
   c. Protons
   d. Neutrons

8. What is different between the isotopes of an atom?
   a. The number of protons
   b. The number of orbitals
   c. The number of neutrons
   d. The location of the nucleus

9. How are elements with similar chemical properties sorted on the Periodic Table?
   a. By rows
   b. By columns
   c. In the top row only
   d. Randomly throughout the table

10. Which type of reaction is represented by the following equation: A + B → C?
    a. Decomposition
    b. Combustion
    c. Enzymatic
    d. Combination

11. How do catalysts work to increase the rate of a reaction?
    a. By decreasing the number of reactants
    b. By lowering the activation energy required to drive the reaction forward
    c. By increasing the temperature of the reaction environment
    d. By decreasing the number of products that are formed

12. Which of the following is NOT a step in solving a stoichiometry problem?
    a. Find the number of total products.
    b. Balance the equation.
    c. Add a new reactant to the equation.
    d. Calculate the desired information regarding molar mass or percent yield.

13. What is the molar mass of a substance?
    a. The mass of one mole of the substance
    b. The mass of ten molecules of the substance
    c. The number of protons in the substance
    d. The number of atoms in the substance

14. Which of the following is one main type of transfer that occurs in redox reactions?
    a. Transfer of carbon
    b. Transfer of hydrogen
    c. Transfer of nitrogen
    d. Transfer of sulfur

15. Which of the following descriptions characterizes an oxidative agent in a redox reaction?
    a. When it gains a hydrogen
    b. When it loses an oxygen
    c. When it gains one or more electrons
    d. When it gains a carbon

16. What is the sum of the oxidation numbers of all the atoms in a neutral compound?
  a. 1
  b. −1
  c. 2
  d. 0

17. What color does red litmus paper turn if the solution is a base?
  a. Blue
  b. Green
  c. Stays red
  d. Purple

18. What number on the pH scale indicates a neutral solution?
  a. 13
  b. 8
  c. 7
  d. 2

19. Which of the following compounds is an example of a strong base?
  a. HCl
  b. HNO_3
  c. HBr
  d. NaOH

20. What does the half-life of a substance calculate?
  a. The time it takes for the substance to completely decay
  b. The time it takes for the substance to reach the halfway point of its lifespan
  c. The number of neutrons in the isotope of the substance
  d. The current age of the substance

21. Which type of nuclear radioactive decay emits two protons and two neutrons from its nucleus?
  a. Gamma
  b. Beta
  c. Alpha
  d. Uranium

22. Which of the following is NOT one of the three elements that can begin a naturally occurring radioactive decay series?
  a. Uranium-235
  b. Thorium
  c. Uranium-238
  d. Neptunium

23. How can radiation help with medical treatments?
  a. A short exposure can be targeted at a specific area to knock out harmful cells, such as in cancer.
  b. It can break chemical bonds in DNA.
  c. It can diminish the body's ability to produce cells.
  d. It can mutate cells.

24. Palmitoleic acid is a fatty acid that is liquid at room temperature. Which of the following is likely true?
   a. Palmitoleic acid is a saturated fat.
   b. Palmitoleic acid contains at least one double bond.
   c. Palmitoleic acid is a steroid.
   d. Palmitoleic acid is hydrophilic.

25. Which of the following is an essential amino acid?
   a. Glutamine
   b. Alanine
   c. Leucine
   d. Asparagine

For questions 26–30:

Atoms of a chemical element, or radioactive isotope, naturally go through a process of decay called radioactive decay. Through this process, the atom decays into another element by emitting alpha particles, beta particles, and gamma rays. This process alters the composition of the atom's nucleus until it reaches a stable state. The amount of time it takes for half (50 percent) of the atoms in a sample to decay is referred to as half-life. The figure below shows the decay of Radon 222 into Polonium 218 and other decay products:

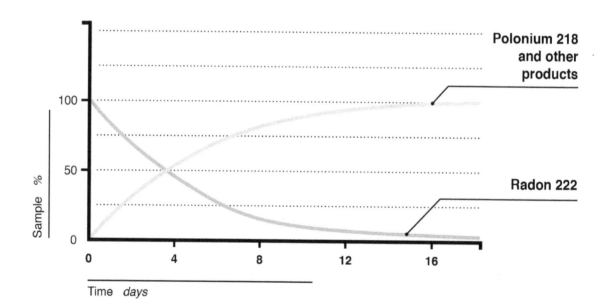

The figure below shows the decay from Mercury 206 into Thallium 206 into Lead 206:

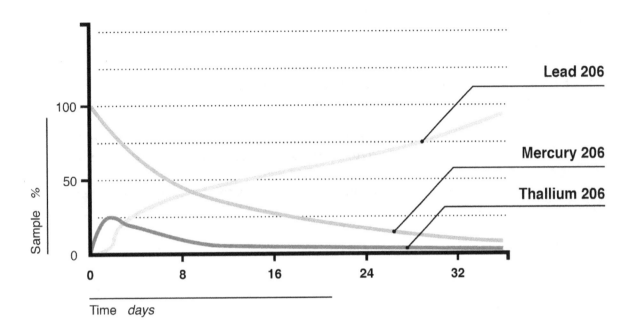

The table below displays the decay products and associated energy million electron volts (MeV) and the type of particle emitted with the decay:

Isotope Particle	Decay Product	Energy (MeV)	Decay Type
Radon 222	Polonium 218	6.190	Alpha
Lead 210	Mercury 206	2.992	Alpha
Mercury 206	Thallium 206	0.912	Beta
Thallium 206	Lead 206	0.813	Beta

26. What is the approximate half-life of Radon 222?
    a. 16 days
    b. 12 days
    c. 4 days
    d. 2 days

27. Which statement is true?
    a. Radioactive decay products are all unstable.
    b. Radioactive decay never occurs naturally.
    c. Radioactive decay is a natural process.
    d. Radioactive decay occurs in half of a sample.

28. Which relationship can be determined from the decay energy and the type of decay particle?
    a. Beta particles have higher decay energies.
    b. Alpha and beta particles have similar decay energies.
    c. Alpha particles have higher decay energies.
    d. There is no relationship between particles and decay energies.

29. When do Radon 222 and Polonium 218 have approximately the same number of atoms remaining?
   a. Day 16
   b. Day 8
   c. Day 4
   d. Day 2

30. Which of the following best describes the Mercury 206 curve in Figure 2?
   a. The rate of decay is a linear function because the number of atoms converting to other elements is constant.
   b. The rate of decay occurs quickly at first, then slows as the number of atoms is reduced.
   c. The rate of decay occurs slowly at first, then speeds up as the number of atoms converting increases.
   d. The rate of decay is sinusoidal because the number of atoms converting to other elements constantly goes up and down.

Answer Explanations

1. A: Physical properties of substances are those that can be observed without changing that substance's chemical composition, such as odor, color, density, and hardness. Reactivity, flammability, and toxicity are all chemical properties of substances. They describe the way in which a substance may change into a different substance. They cannot be observed from the surface.

2. B: Solids have molecules that are packed together tightly and cannot move within their substance. Crystalline solids have atoms or molecules that are arranged symmetrically, making all of the bonds of even strength. When they are broken, they break along a plane of molecules, creating a straight edge. Amorphous solids do not have the symmetrical makeup of crystalline solids. They do not break evenly. Gases and liquids both have molecules that move around freely.

3. A: Chemical reactions are processes that involve the changing of one set of substances to a different set of substances. To accomplish this, the bonds between the atoms in the molecules of the original substances need to be broken. The atoms are rearranged, and new bonds are formed to make the new set of substances. Combination reactions involve two or more reactants becoming one product. Decomposition reactions involve one reactant becoming two or more products. Combustion reactions involve the use of oxygen as a reactant and generally include the burning of a substance. Choices *C* and *D* are not discussed as specific reaction types.

4. A: Scientific notation is a useful system for representing numbers that are very large or very small and cannot be written out without having multiple zeros behind a number in the case of large numbers, or behind a decimal point in the case of small numbers. Any number can be written in scientific notation—there are no restrictions on the digits that comprise the number, as suggested in Choice *B*. While scientific notation is often useful in scientific experiments, it is not used exclusively in this context nor is it mandatory in experiments. For example, if the mass of a substance is measured to be 3.5 g, the investigator would likely report this value rather than convert it to scientific notation (in this case, the number of significant figures is more important). Therefore, Choice *C* is incorrect. Scientific notation is most helpful for numbers larger than 100 or much smaller than 0, making Choice *D* incorrect.

5. C: The metric system uses a base of ten between its units of measure. A centimeter is 1/100 times of the base. Ten-fold greater than that would be 1/10 times of the base, which is a decimeter. A millimeter, Choice *A*, is 10-fold smaller than a centimeter at 1/1000 times of the base. A foot, Choice *B*, is part of the English Standard System and does not have a straightforward comparison to a centimeter. A kilometer, Choice *D*, is 1000 times the base and 100,000-fold greater than a centimeter.

6. D: Water boils at 100 °C, which is equivalent to 212 °F. Water freezes at 0 °C, which is equivalent to 32 °F, Choices *A* and *B*. The temperature of the human body is 98.6 °F, Choice *C*.

7. B: The nucleus contains the protons and neutrons of the atom. Together, they make up 99 percent of the atom's mass. Electrons, Choice *A*, are found in the orbitals surrounding the nucleus and do not have as much mass as the protons or neutrons. Protons and neutrons, Choices *C* and *D*, have similar masses, but neither makes up 99 percent of the atom's mass alone.

8. C: The total number of protons and neutrons in an atom is the atom's mass number. The number of protons in an atom is the atomic number. If an atom has a variation in the number of neutrons, the atom's mass number changes, but the atomic number remains the same. This variation creates isotopes of the atom with the same atomic number. The number of protons, Choice *A*, is unique for each atom and does not change. The number of orbitals and location of the nucleus remain the same for atoms; therefore, Choices *B* and *D* are incorrect.

9. B: The columns of the periodic table have elements with similar chemical properties, such as appearance and reactivity. The elements in rows, Choice *A*, are arranged with similar electron valance configurations. Moving from left to right and top to bottom, the elements are arranged according to atomic number. Therefore, the top row contains elements with similar numbers of protons, making Choice *C* incorrect. The periodic table is highly organized, so similar elements are grouped together and are not randomly scattered throughout the table; thus, Choice *D* is incorrect.

10. D: The equation A + B → C represents a combination reaction because two reactants are being combined to form one larger product. Decomposition reactions, Choice *A*, are represented as C → B + A, where one larger reactant is broken into two smaller products. Combustion reactions, Choice *B*, always involve oxygen gas as a reactant. Although most reactions involve enzymes, this equation does not specify whether an enzyme is involved, so Choice *C* is incorrect.

11. B: The activation energy is the amount of energy that is required for a reaction to move forward and change the reactants into products. Catalysts decrease the amount of energy that needs to be generated to drive the reaction to happen, so they lower the activation energy of the reaction. The number of reactants and products, Choices *A* and *D*, remain the same in catalytic reactions. Although increasing temperature can increase the rate of a reaction, it is not how catalysts work; thus, Choice *C* is incorrect.

12. C: Stoichiometry problems involve solving a chemical equation as written without adding any more reactants to the mix. The first step is to balance the equation, Choice *B*. The next step is to find the total number of products, Choice *A*. The last step is to calculate the information that is needed to find the ratios of reactants to obtain the products, Choice *D*.

13. A: The molar mass of a substance is equivalent to the mass of one mole of the substance. It can be found on the periodic table for individual elements and is listed as the atomic mass unit. For example, the molar mass of carbon is 12.01 g/mol. One mole is equivalent to 6.02×10^{23} molecules of a substance, not only ten molecules; therefore, Choice *B* is incorrect. The number of protons is the atomic number of an element, so Choice *C* is incorrect. The number of atoms is unrelated to the molar mass; thus, Choice *D* is incorrect.

14. B: Redox reactions are chemical reactions that involve one species of the reactants being oxidized and another species of the reactants being reduced. The transferring of hydrogen between reactants is one type of redox reaction. Another type involves the transferring of oxygen between reactants, and the third type involves the transferring of electrons between the reactants. Carbon, nitrogen, and sulfur, Choices *A, C,* and *D,* do not drive redox reactions.

15. C: A reactant is an oxidative agent when it gains electrons, gains an oxygen, or loses a hydrogen. Choices *A* and *B* describe the opposite situations. Carbon is not involved in the transfer of electrons, or when hydrogen acts as a proton, in redox reactions. Therefore, Choice *D* is incorrect.

16. D: The oxidation number of a compound is the charge that the compound would have if it was composed of ions. Neutral compounds do not have a charge, so their oxidation number is 0. The oxidation number of hydrogen is 1, but it is –1 when it is combined with elements that are not as electronegative. Group 2 elements in a compound have an oxidation number of 2. Thus, Choices *A, B,* and *C* are incorrect.

17. A: Red litmus paper will turn blue if the solution being tested is a base. If the solution is neutral or acidic, the paper will stay red, Choice *C*. Red litmus paper does not turn green or purple, so Choices *B* and *D* do not apply in this situation.

18. C: The pH scale goes from 0 to 14. A neutral solution falls right in the middle of the scale at 7. Choice *A*, a value of 13, indicates a strong base. Choice *B*, a value of 8, indicates a solution that is weakly basic. Choice *D*, a value of 2, indicates a strong acid.

19. D: A strong base dissociates completely and forms the anion OH⁻. All bases include a hydroxide group (OH) in their formula, but not all basic compounds will dissociate completely; only strong bases dissociate completely into ions. Choices *A*, *B*, and *C* all represent strong acids and have a hydrogen atom, which is always present in acidic compounds.

20. B: The nuclei of radioactive substances emit particles and energy in the process of radioactive decay. The half-life of a substance refers to the length of time for the nuclei in half of the atoms in a substance to completely decay, so this is essentially indicative of when half of the "lifetime" of the substance (in terms of its existence) has elapsed. Thus, Choice *B* is correct. It is impossible to predict when an atom will completely decay, so Choice *A* is wrong. Isotopes have different numbers of neutrons than the atoms they are derived from, but this is unrelated to calculation of half-life, so Choice *C* is incorrect. The half-life is a specific calculation for the time it takes for the nuclei in atoms of a radioactive substance to have undergone radioactive decay and does not calculate the current age of the atom; therefore, Choice *D* is incorrect.

21. C: Alpha nuclear decay involves that atom emitting two protons and two neutrons from its nucleus. Since protons are emitted from the nucleus, the atom becomes a different element with a new atomic number. Gamma nuclear decay, Choice *A*, does not change the mass or charge of an atom. Beta nuclear decay, Choice *B*, causes an atom to turn a neutron into a proton and an electron. The increase in proton and electron count causes a new element to be formed. Uranium decay, Choice *D*, is not a type of radioactive decay.

22. D: Neptunium is an artificially-made element that starts an artificial radioactive decay series. The only three naturally-occurring elements that can start a naturally-occurring radioactive decay series are uranium-235, thorium, and uranium-238, which are Choices *A*, *B*, and *C*. These elements decay into a series of other naturally-occurring elements until they end up as a more stable element.

23. A: Radiation can be both helpful and harmful in medical treatments. Short exposures to radiation can knock out harmful cancer cells. Radioactive tracers can also be used to detect how a system in the body is working. Breaking the chemical bonds of DNA, Choice *B*, is harmful to the body. If the body can no longer produce cells, Choice *C*, damaged cells cannot be replaced, and the body's health will decline. Mutations to the cells, Choice *D*, can be harmful to the body as well.

24. B: Palmitoleic acid is liquid at room temperature, which is characteristic of an unsaturated fatty acid. Unsaturated fats contain at least one double bond, which causes a kink in the fatty acid chain. This kink prevents the fatty acid chains from packing together tightly, and this looser arrangement causes most unsaturated fats to be liquid at room temperature. Palmitoleic acid is not a steroid, which consist of a four-ring structure containing one ring of five carbons and three rings of six carbons. Like most fats, palmitoleic acid is hydrophobic, not hydrophilic, so Choice *D* is incorrect.

25. C: Leucine is an essential amino acid. The essential amino acids must be consumed for proper health and function because the body cannot synthesize them. Glutamine, Choice *A*, is a conditional amino acid.

The human body can generally produce conditional amino acids but may not be able to during times of stress or illness. Alanine and asparagine, Choices *B* and *D*, are nonessential amino acids.

26. C: According to Figure 1, 50 percent of the sample remains after approximately four days. This is where the graph lines up with 50 percent on the y-axis and drops down to four days on the x-axis.

27. C: As stated in the example, radioactive decay is a natural process that happens spontaneously when atoms of one element decay into another element. Choice *A* is incorrect because decay occurs until the atoms in the sample reach a stable state. It is not limited to only half of the atoms; therefore, Choice *D* is incorrect.

28. C: According to Table 1, the higher energy emissions were matched with the alpha particle emissions. The alpha particles had higher emissions than the beta particles in all instances listed; there was a relationship between the emission energies and the types of particles emitted, so Choice *D* is incorrect.

29. C: According to Figure 1, the two lines intersect with each other at approximately Day 4.

30. B: The rate of decay occurs quickly at first, then slows as the number of Mercury 206 atoms is reduced.

Anatomy and Physiology

General Terminology

Anatomy is the study of external and internal body parts and structures, and their physical relationships to each other. **Physiology** is the study of the function of living organisms and their body parts. The human body is made up of different types of *cells* that join together to form tissues, which then form together to create organs. Although there are trillions of cells in the human body, there are only about two hundred different types of cells. *Organs* provide functions for the body that are vital for sustaining life. There are four primary types of *tissue* found in the human body: epithelial, connective, muscle, and neural. Each tissue type has specific characteristics that enable organs and organ systems to function properly. *Epithelial tissue* includes epithelia and glands. *Epithelia* are the layers of cells that cover exposed surfaces and line internal cavities and passageways. *Glands* are structures that are involved in secretion of fluids. Epithelia do not contain blood vessels and can often regenerate quickly to replace dead and damaged cells. *Connective tissue* fills internal spaces and is never exposed to the outside of the body. It provides structural support for the body and stores energy. This type of tissue is also a protective barrier for delicate organs and for the body against microorganisms. *Muscle tissue* has characteristics that make it specialized for contraction, which is the force that produces movement in the body. It also helps the body maintain posture and is responsible for controlling body temperature. *Neural tissue* conducts electrical impulses, which help send information and instructions throughout the body. Most of it is concentrated in the brain and spinal cord.

Histology

Histology is the study of cells and tissues on a microscopic level. Live cells and tissue can be cultured and maintained in a laboratory for research purposes. When researchers want to observe them at certain stages of their life cycle or at different times, the cells or tissue samples can be fixed, sectioned, stained, and then mounted onto a microscope slide. Their anatomy can then be visualized under different types of microscopes depending on which features are being looked at and what type of stain was used. Histopathology is a specialized area of histology that focuses on the study of diseased tissue. Studying the differences between normal and diseased tissue is a critical part of diagnosing and treating diseases such as cancer.

The first step in preparing a sample for histological analysis is to fix the sample. Fixation preserves the tissue from degradation and maintains the structure of cells, including subcellular components, such as cell organelles. If the sample will be viewed under a light microscope, the most common fixative that is used is a 4% formaldehyde solution in phosphate buffered saline (PBS). For electron microscopes, samples are usually fixed in a 2.5% glutaraldehyde solution in PBS. The fixatives work by irreversibly cross-linking proteins with the sample. Since the tissue sample must be very hard before it can be sectioned and placed on a microscope slide, the tissue must then be dehydrated to remove any water in the sample. It is generally washed through a series of increasingly concentrated ethanol baths, followed by a xylene rinse to remove the ethanol. Then, the samples are placed in molten paraffin wax to replace the xylene for light microscope samples. Electron microscope samples use a resin material instead since they provide harder samples. After the internal embedding is complete, the samples are externally embedded in a larger mold and hardened. Once the embedded samples are hard enough, they can be sectioned using a microtome. Samples for light microscopy are cut using a steel knife in the microtome to produce sections that are four micrometers thick. These sections can be mounted individually on glass microscope slides. Samples for electron microscopy must be cut much thinner. They are cut using a diamond knife in an ultramicrotome to produce sections that are only fifty nanometers thick. These samples are mounted onto a copper grid. The embedded samples can be cut in any direction, depending on what the researcher is looking to see. Lastly, the samples that are mounted onto the slides can be stained. Many different types of stains can be used to elucidate specific features of the sample. Different stains can selectively highlight different parts of the cell. The most common type of stain used in histology is hematoxylin and eosin staining. The hematoxylin stains the nuclei of cells blue and the eosin stains the cytoplasm of cells pink.

Histological samples can also be processed by freezing. This process is often used for oncology samples because of its speed, but it produces a lower quality histology sample. With frozen fixation, the tissue sample is embedded in a gel material and then placed on a metal disk and then frozen rapidly to -20 to -30 °C. The sample becomes very hard and can then be sliced under refrigeration using a cryostat machine. The thin layers can then be mounted onto microscope slides.

Mitosis and Meiosis

Mitosis

Mitosis is a process that cells use to reproduce exact copies of themselves. It helps organisms to grow themselves and their population. Single-celled organisms can only use mitosis to reproduce (this is considered asexual reproduction). Multicellular organisms use mitosis to reproduce all cells except for their germ cells, which are reproduced by meiosis. Mitosis is a five-stage process that divides the genetic material in the nucleus of the cells. The first stage, *prophase*, is when the mitotic spindles begin to form. The spindles comprise centrosomes and microtubules. The microtubules lengthen and the centromeres move towards opposite ends of the cell. Two identical chromosomes join together. Next, during *prometaphase*, the chromosome pairs develop a kinetochore, which is a specialized protein that joins them together, and become further condensed. The nuclear envelope starts to break down.

In *metaphase*, the microtubules stretch across the cell and the centrosomes have reached opposite ends of the cell. The chromosomes align in the middle of the cell, along the metaphase plate, which is a plane that runs exactly between the two centrosomes. As mitosis begins to reach completion, during the penultimate stage of *anaphase*, the chromosome pairs break apart, forming two fully developed, independent chromosomes. One set of chromosomes moves to each end of the cell. The cell elongates while the microtubules shorten towards opposite ends of the cell.

Telophase is the final stage of mitosis. Two nuclei form at each end of the cell and a nuclear envelope begins to form around each nucleus. The chromosomes become less condensed and the microtubules are broken down. The cytoplasm is divided by a process called *cytokinesis*, which marks the end of mitosis.

The process of mitosis

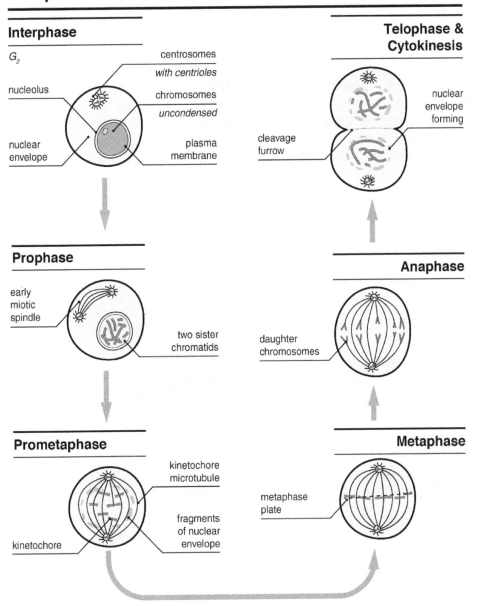

Meiosis

Unlike mitosis, **meiosis** produces daughter cells that are not identical to the parent cells. In addition, the parent cell is diploid and the daughter cells are haploid, which means that the parent cell has twice as many chromosomes as the daughter cells it produces. At the end of meiosis, four daughter cells are produced, whereas in mitosis, two daughter cells are produced. Meiosis follows the same stages as mitosis; however, they occur twice—once during meiosis I and again during meiosis II. The parent cell has two sets of chromosomes, set A and set B. One set comes from the germ cell from each parent, which in the case of humans, is the sperm and the egg. During prophase I, each chromosome set duplicates itself exactly and then pairs up with its identical chromosome so that they are matched up along their entire lengths. A protein structure called the synaptonemal complex holds the pairs together. Between prophase I and metaphase I, a process called *crossing over* occurs. This is when the genes on the chromosomes are traded between each other, producing chromosomes that are no longer identical to the parent chromosomes. The synaptonemal complex helps with the exchange of genes during this process. The areas where the paired chromosomes are linked together during crossing over, called chiasmata, can be visualized under a microscope. Chiasmata are responsible for holding the new remixed chromosomes together after the synaptonemal complex breaks down. Once crossing over is complete, the mitotic spindles take hold of the chromosomes and move them towards the center of the cell. The two homologues of the same chromosome pairs attach to spindles that are attached to opposite poles of the cell. In anaphase I, the homologues are pulled apart in opposite directions and in telophase I, the chromosomes have reached the opposite poles. The parent cell then splits into two cells. Next, in meiosis II, the intermediate daughter cells divide again. The chromosomes are not duplicated, however. During this stage, the chromosome pairs are separated from each other into four haploid cells, each with one set of chromosomes.

The process of mitosis

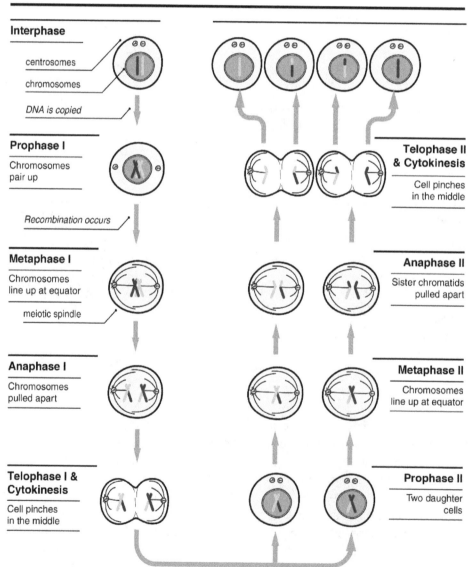

Skin

The **integumentary system** protects the body from damage from the outside. It consists of skin and its appendages, including hair, nails, and sweat glands. This system functions as a cushion, a waterproof layer, a temperature regulator, and a protectant of the deeper tissues within the body. It also excretes waste from the body. The skin is the largest organ of the human body, consisting of two layers called the epidermis and the dermis. The *epidermis* can be classified as thick or thin. Most of the body is covered with thin skin, but areas such as the palm of the hands are covered with thick skin. The epidermis is responsible for synthesizing vitamin D when exposed to UV rays. Vitamin D is essential to the body for the processes of calcium and phosphorus absorption, which maintain healthy bones. The *dermis* lies under the epidermis and consists of a superficial papillary layer and a deeper reticular layer. The *papillary layer* is made up of loose connective tissue and contains capillaries and the axons of sensory neurons. The *reticular layer* is a meshwork of tightly packed irregular connective tissue and contains blood vessels, hair follicles, nerves, sweat glands, and sebaceous glands.

The three major functions of skin are protection, regulation, and sensation. Skin acts as a barrier and protects the body from mechanical impacts, variations in temperature, microorganisms, and chemicals. It regulates body temperature, peripheral circulation, and fluid balance by secreting sweat. It also contains a large network of nerve cells that relay changes in the external environment to the body.

Hair serves many functions for the human body. It provides sensation, protects against heat loss, and filters air that is taken in through the nose. Nails provide a hard layer of protection over soft skin. Sweat glands and sebaceous glands are two important *exocrine glands* found in the skin. *Sweat glands* regulate temperature and remove bodily waste by secreting water, nitrogenous waste, and sodium salts to the surface of the body. *Sebaceous glands* secrete *sebum*, which is an oily mixture of lipids and proteins. Sebum protects the skin from water loss and bacterial and fungal infections.

Skeletal System

The adult **skeletal system** consists of the 206 bones that make up the skeleton, as well as the cartilage, ligaments, and other connective tissues that stabilize them. Babies are born with roughly three hundred bones, some of which fuse together during growth. *Bone* is made up of collagen fibers and mineral salts (mainly calcium and phosphorus). The mineral salts are strong but brittle, and the collagen fibers are weak but flexible, so the combination makes bone very resistant to shattering.

There are two types of bone: compact and spongy. *Compact bone,* also called cortical bone, is dense with a matrix filled with organic substances and inorganic salts. There are only tiny spaces left between these materials for the *osteocytes,* or bone cells, to fit into. *Spongy bone,* in contrast to compact bone, is lightweight and porous. Also called cancellous bone, spongy bone covers the outside of the bone and gives it a shiny, white appearance. It has a branching network of parallel lamellae called *trabeculae.* Although spongy bone forms an open framework around the compact bone, it is still quite strong. Different bones have different ratios of compact to spongy bone depending on their function.

The outside of the bone is covered by a *periosteum,* which has four major functions. It isolates and protects bones from the surrounding tissue, provides a place for attachment of the circulatory and nervous system structures, participates in growth and repair of the bone, and attaches the bone to the deep fascia. An *endosteum* is found inside the bone; it covers the trabeculae of the spongy bone and lines the inner surfaces of the central canals.

One of the major functions of the skeletal system is to provide structural support for the entire body. It provides a framework for the soft tissues and organs to attach to. The skeletal system also provides a reserve of important nutrients, such as calcium and lipids. Normal concentrations of calcium and phosphorus in body fluids are partly maintained by the calcium salts stored in bone. Lipids that are stored in yellow bone marrow can be used as a source of energy. Yellow bone marrow also produces some white blood cells. Red bone marrow produces red blood cells, most white blood cells, and platelets that circulate in the blood. Certain groups of bones form protective barriers around delicate organs. The ribs, for example, protect the heart and lungs, the skull encloses the brain, and the vertebrae cover the spinal cord.

Muscular System

The **neuromuscular, or muscular, system** is composed of all of the muscles in the human body and the nerves that control them. Every movement that the body makes is controlled by the brain. There are approximately seven hundred muscles in the body. There are three types of muscle tissue in the body. *Skeletal muscle tissue* is attached to the bones of the skeletal system and makes up half of the body's weight. It pulls on the bones of the skeleton and causes body movement. *Cardiac muscle tissue* helps to pump blood through veins and arteries. Lastly, *smooth muscle tissue* helps to move fluids and solids along the digestive tract, and also contributes to movement in other body systems.

An important characteristic of all types of muscle is that they are *excitable*, which means that they respond to electrical stimuli. *Neurons*, or nerve cells, are the main cells responsible for transferring and processing information between the brain and other parts of the body. *Neuroglia* are cells that support the neurons by providing a framework around them and isolating them from the surrounding environment.

Nervous System

The nervous system is made up of the **central nervous system (CNS)** and the **peripheral nervous system (PNS)**. The CNS includes the brain and the spinal cord, while the PNS includes the rest of the neural tissue that is not included in the CNS. The CNS is responsible for processing and coordinating sensory data and motor commands. The PNS, on the other hand, is responsible for relaying sensory information and motor commands between the CNS and peripheral tissues and systems. The PNS has two subdivisions, known as the afferent and efferent divisions. The *afferent division* relays sensory information to the CNS and supplies information from the skin and joints about the body's sensation and balance. The *efferent division* transmits motor commands to muscles and glands. The efferent division consists of the *somatic nervous system (SNS)*, which controls skeletal muscle contractions and allows the brain to control body movement, and the *autonomic nervous system (ANS)*, which regulates activity of smooth muscle, cardiac muscle, and glands, and allows the brain to control heart rate, blood pressure, and body temperature.

Endocrine System

The **endocrine system** is made up of ductless tissues and glands, and is responsible for hormone secretion into either the blood or the interstitial fluid of the human body. *Hormones* are chemical substances that change the metabolic activity of tissues and organs. *Interstitial fluid* is the solution that surrounds tissue cells within the body. This system works closely with the nervous system to regulate the physiological activities of the other systems of the body in order to maintain homeostasis. While the nervous system provides quick, short-term responses to stimuli, the endocrine system acts by releasing hormones into the bloodstream, which then are distributed to the whole body. The response is slow but long-lasting, ranging from a few hours to even a few weeks. While regular metabolic reactions are controlled by enzymes, hormones can change the type, activity, or quantity of the enzymes involved in the reaction. They can regulate development and growth, metabolism, mood, and body temperature, among many other things. Often very small amounts of a hormone will lead to large changes in the body.

There are eight major glands in the endocrine system, each with its own specific function. They are described below.

- Hypothalamus: This gland is a part of the brain. It connects the nervous system to the endocrine system via the pituitary gland and plays an important role in regulating endocrine organs.

- Pituitary gland: This pea-sized gland is found at the bottom of the hypothalamus. It releases hormones that regulate growth, blood pressure, certain functions of the reproductive sex organs, and pain relief, among other things. It also plays an important role in regulating the function of other endocrine glands.

- Thyroid gland: This gland releases hormones that are important for metabolism, growth and development, temperature regulation, and brain development during infancy and childhood. Thyroid hormones also monitor the amount of circulating calcium in the body.

- Parathyroid glands: These are four pea-sized glands located on the posterior surface of the thyroid. The main hormone that is secreted is called parathyroid hormone (PTH); it helps with the thyroid's regulation of calcium in the body.

- Thymus gland: This gland is located in the chest cavity, embedded in connective tissue. It produces several hormones that are important for development and maintenance of normal immunological defenses.

- Adrenal glands: One adrenal gland is attached to the top of each kidney. Its major function is to aid in the management of stress.

- Pancreas: This gland produces hormones that regulate blood sugar levels in the body.

- Pineal gland: The pineal gland secretes the hormone melatonin, which can slow the maturation of sperm, oocytes, and reproductive organs. Melatonin also regulates the body's circadian rhythm, which is the natural awake-asleep cycles.

Circulatory System

The **cardiovascular system** is composed of the heart and blood vessels. The *heart*, which is the main organ of the cardiovascular system, acts as a pump and circulates blood throughout the body. Gases, nutrients, and waste are constantly exchanged between the circulating blood and interstitial fluid, keeping tissues and organs alive and healthy. The heart is located behind the sternum, on the left side, in the front of the chest. The heart wall is made up of three distinct layers. The outer layer, called the *epicardium*, is a serous membrane that is also known as the *visceral pericardium*. The middle layer is called the *myocardium* and contains connective tissue, blood vessels, and nerves within its layers of cardiac muscle tissue. The inner layer is called the *endocardium*, and is made up of a simple squamous epithelium. It includes the heart valves and is continuous with the endothelium of the attached blood vessels. The heart has four chambers: the *right atrium*, the *right ventricle*, the *left atrium*, and the *left ventricle*. The atrium and ventricle on the same side of the heart have an opening between them that is regulated by a valve.

The valve maintains blood flow in only one direction, moving from the atrium to the ventricle, and prevents backflow. The right side of the heart has a *tricuspid valve* (because it has three leaflets) between the chambers, and the left side of the heart has a *bicuspid valve* (with two leaflets) between the chambers, also called the *mitral valve*. Oxygen-poor blood from the body enters the right atrium and is pumped into the right ventricle. The blood then enters the pulmonary trunk and flows into the pulmonary arteries, where it can become re-oxygenated. Oxygen-rich blood from the lungs then flows into the left atrium, passes into the left ventricle, enters the aorta, and gets pumped to the rest of the body.

Blood is an important vehicle for transport of oxygen, nutrients, and hormones throughout the body. It is composed of plasma and formed elements, which include red blood cells (RBCs), white blood cells (WBCs), and platelets. *Plasma* is the liquid matrix of the blood and contains dissolved proteins. *RBCs* contain hemoglobin, which carries oxygen through the blood. Red blood cells also transport carbon dioxide. *WBCs* are part of the immune system and help fight off diseases. *Platelets* contain enzymes and other factors that help with blood clotting. Blood circulates throughout the body in vessels called arteries, veins, and capillaries. These vessels are muscular tubes that allow gas exchange to occur. *Arteries* carry oxygen-rich blood from the heart to the other tissues of the body. *Veins* collect oxygen-depleted blood from tissues and organs and return it back to the heart. *Capillaries* are the smallest of the blood vessels and do not function individually; instead, they work together in a unit called a *capillary bed*. Their thin walls are only one cell layer in thickness, so capillaries are the primary site of gas exchange between the blood and tissues.

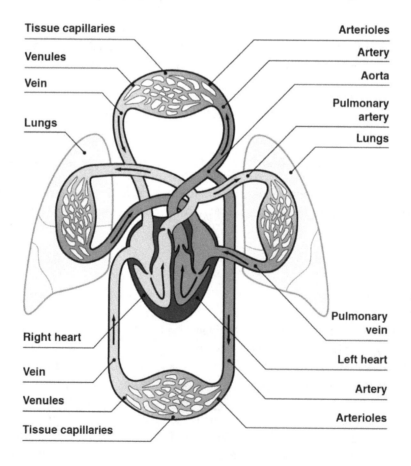

Respiratory System

The **respiratory system** is responsible for gas exchange between air and the blood, mainly via the act of breathing. It is divided into two sections: the upper respiratory system and the lower respiratory system. The *upper respiratory system* includes the nose, the nasal cavity and sinuses, and the pharynx, while the *lower respiratory system* includes the larynx (voice box), the trachea (windpipe), the small passageways leading to the lungs, and the lungs. The upper respiratory system is responsible for filtering, warming, and humidifying the air that gets passed to the lower respiratory system, protecting the lower respiratory system's more delicate tissue surfaces.

The human body has two lungs, each having its own distinct characteristics. The *right lung* is divided into three lobes (superior, middle, and inferior), and the *left lung* is divided into two lobes (superior and inferior). The left lung is thought to be smaller than the right lung because it shares space in the chest cavity with the heart. Together, the lungs contain approximately fifteen hundred miles of airway passages, which are the site of gas exchange during the act of breathing. When a breath of air is inhaled, oxygen enters the nose or mouth and passes into the sinuses, which is where the temperature and humidity of the air get regulated. The air then passes into the trachea and is filtered. From there, it travels into the bronchi and reaches the lungs. Bronchi are lined with cilia and mucus that collect dust and germs along the way. Within the lungs, oxygen and carbon dioxide are exchanged between the air in the *alveoli*, thin sacs in the lungs, and the blood in the *pulmonary capillaries*, a type of blood vessel in the lungs. Oxygen-rich blood returns to the heart and gets pumped through the systemic circuit. Carbon dioxide-rich air is exhaled from the body.

The respiratory system has many important functions in the body. Most importantly, it provides a large area for gas exchange between the air and the circulating blood. It protects the delicate respiratory surfaces from environmental variations and defends them against pathogens. It is responsible for producing the sounds that the body makes for speaking and singing, as well as for nonverbal communication. It also helps regulate blood volume, blood pressure, and the pH of blood.

Respiratory System

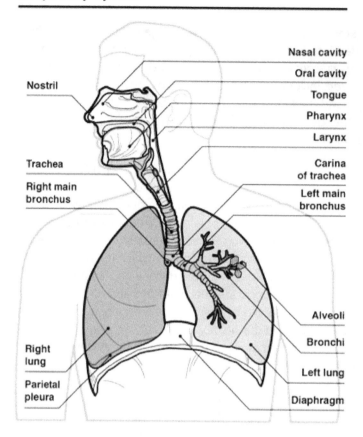

Nasal cavity
Oral cavity
Tongue
Pharynx
Larynx
Carina of trachea
Left main bronchus
Alveoli
Bronchi
Left lung
Diaphragm

Nostril
Trachea
Right main bronchus
Right lung
Parietal pleura

Digestive System

The **gastrointestinal system** is a group of organs that work together to fuel the body by transforming food and liquids into energy. After food is ingested, it passes through the *alimentary canal*, or *GI tract*, which consists of the mouth, pharynx, esophagus, stomach, small intestine, and large intestine. Each organ has a specific function to aid in digestion. The *stomach* stores food so that the body has time to digest large meals. It secretes enzymes and acids and also helps with mechanical processing through *peristalsis* or muscular contractions. The *small intestine* is a thin tube that is approximately ten feet long. It secretes enzymes and has many folds that increase its surface area to allow for maximum absorption of nutrients from the digested food. The *large intestine* is a long, thick tube that is about five feet in length. It absorbs water from the digested food and transports waste to be excreted from the body. It also contains symbiotic bacteria that break down the waste products even further, allowing for any additional nutrients, mainly in the form of vitamins and minerals, to be absorbed.

In addition to these main organs, the gastrointestinal system has a few accessory organs that help break down food without having the food or liquid pass directly through them. The *liver* produces and secretes *bile*, which is important for the digestion of lipids. It also plays a large role in the regulation of circulating levels of carbohydrates, amino acids, and lipids in the body. Excess nutrients are removed by the liver and deficiencies are corrected with its stored nutrients, including the fat-soluble vitamins (A, E, D, and K), vitamin B12, iron, and copper. The *gallbladder* is responsible for storing and concentrating bile before it gets secreted into the small intestine. The *pancreas* secretes buffers and digestive enzymes. It contains specific enzymes for each type of food molecule, such as *amylases* for carbohydrates, *lipases* for lipids, and *proteases* for proteins.

Listed below are seven main steps involved in the transformation of food as it travels through the gastrointestinal system:

1. Ingestion: Food and liquids enter the alimentary canal through the mouth.

2. Mechanical processing: Food is torn up and mashed by the teeth and swirled around by the tongue to facilitate swallowing.

3. Digestion: Chemicals and enzymes break down complex molecules, such as sugars, lipids, and proteins, into smaller molecules that can be absorbed by the digestive epithelium.

4. Secretion: Most of the acids, buffers, and enzymes that aid in digestion are secreted by the accessory organs, but some are provided by the digestive tract.

5. Absorption: Vitamins, electrolytes, organic molecules, and water are absorbed by the digestive epithelium and moved to the interstitial fluid of the digestive tract.

6. Compaction: Indigestible materials and organic wastes are dehydrated and compacted before eliminated from the body.

7. Excretion: Waste products are secreted into the digestive tract.

Gastrointestinal System

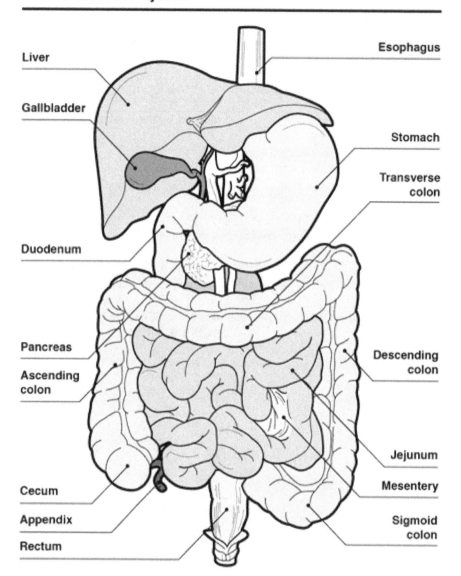

Liver

Gallbladder

Duodenum

Pancreas

Ascending colon

Cecum

Appendix

Rectum

Esophagus

Stomach

Transverse colon

Descending colon

Jejunum

Mesentery

Sigmoid colon

Urinary System

The **genitourinary system** encompasses the reproductive organs and the *urinary system*. They are often grouped together because of their proximity to each other in the body, and, for the male, because of shared pathways. The external male genitalia include the penis, urethra, and scrotum. Both urine and male gametes travel through the urethra within the penis to exit the body. In both the male and female bodies, the urinary system is made up of the kidneys, ureters, urinary bladder, and the urethra. It is the main system responsible for getting rid of the organic waste products, as well as excess water and electrolytes that are generated by the other systems of the body. Regulation of the water and electrolytes also contributes to the maintenance of blood pH.

Under normal circumstances, humans have two functioning *kidneys*, which are the main organs responsible for filtering waste products out of the blood and transferring them to urine. Every day, the kidneys filter approximately 120 to 150 quarts of blood and produce one to two quarts of urine. The kidneys are made up of millions of tiny filtering units called *nephrons*. Nephrons have two parts: a *glomerulus*, which is the filter, and a *tubule*. As blood enters the kidneys, the glomerulus allows for fluid and waste products to pass through it and enter the tubule. Blood cells and large molecules, such as proteins, do not pass through and remain in the blood. The filtered fluid and waste then pass through the tubule, where any final essential minerals can be sent back to the bloodstream. The final product at the end of the tubule is called *urine*. The urine travels through the *ureters* into the *urinary bladder*, which is a hollow, elastic muscular organ. As more and more urine enters the urinary bladder, its walls stretch and become thinner so that there is no significant difference in internal pressure. The urinary bladder stores the urine until the body is ready for urination, at which time, its muscles contract and force the urine through the urethra and out of the body.

Reproductive System

The **reproductive system** is responsible for producing, storing, nourishing, and transporting functional reproductive cells, or *gametes*, in the human body. It includes the reproductive organs, also known as *gonads*, the *reproductive tract*, the accessory glands and organs that secrete fluids into the reproductive tract, and the *perineal structures*, which are the external genitalia. The human male and female reproductive systems are very different from each other.

The male gonads are called *testes*. The testes secrete androgens, mainly testosterone, and produce and store one-half billion *sperms cells*, which are the male gametes, each day. An *androgen* is a steroid hormone that controls the development and maintenance of male characteristics. Once the sperm are mature, they move through a duct system where they are mixed with additional fluids that are secreted by accessory glands, forming a mixture called *semen*. The sperm cells in semen are responsible for fertilization of the female gametes to produce offspring. The male reproductive system has a few accessory organs as well, which are located inside the body. The *prostate gland* and the *seminal vesicles* provide additional fluid that serves as nourishment to the sperm during ejaculation. The *vas deferens* is responsible for transportation of sperm to the urethra. The *bulbourethral glands* produce a lubricating fluid for the urethra that also neutralizes the residual acidity left behind by urine.

The female gonads are called *ovaries*. Ovaries generally produce one immature gamete, or *oocyte*, per month. The ovaries are also responsible for secreting the hormones estrogen and progesterone. When the oocyte is released from the ovary, it travels along the uterine tubes, or *Fallopian tubes*, and then into the *uterus*. The uterus opens into the vagina. When sperm cells enter the vagina, they swim through the uterus. If they fertilize the oocyte, they do so in the Fallopian tubes. The resulting zygote travels down the tube and implants into the uterine wall. The uterus protects and nourishes the developing embryo for nine months until it is ready for the outside environment. If the oocyte is not fertilized, it is released in the menstrual cycle. The *menstrual cycle* usually occurs monthly and involves the shedding of the functional part of the uterine lining. *Mammary glands* are a specialized accessory organ of the female reproductive system. The mammary glands are located in the breast tissue of females. During pregnancy, the glands begin to grow as the cells proliferate in preparation for lactation. After pregnancy, the cells begin to secrete nutrient-filled milk, which is transferred into a duct system and out through the nipple for nourishment of the baby.

HESI A&P Practice Questions

1. How many different types of cells are there in the human body?
    a. Two hundred
    b. One thousand
    c. Ten
    d. Twenty-five

2. What type of tissue provides a protective barrier for delicate organs?
    a. Epithelial
    b. Muscle
    c. Connective
    d. Neural

3. What part of the respiratory system is responsible for regulating the temperature and humidity of the air that comes into the body?
    a. Larynx
    b. Lungs
    c. Trachea
    d. Sinuses

4. Which of the following is true regarding the circulatory system?
    a. Carbon dioxide-rich blood returns to the heart to get pumped through systemic circulation.
    b. The mitral valve prevents backflow of blood from the right ventricle back into the right atrium.
    c. Oxygen-rich blood leave the right ventricle and enters pulmonary circulation.
    d. The bicuspid valve closes after the left ventricle has filled with blood.

5. Which organ is responsible for gas exchange between air and circulating blood?
    a. Nose
    b. Larynx
    c. Lungs
    d. Stomach

6. Which layer of the heart wall contains nerves?
    a. Epicardium
    b. Myocardium
    c. Endocardium
    d. Sternum

7. What is another name for the mitral valve?
    a. Bicuspid valve
    b. Pulmonary valve
    c. Aortic valve
    d. Tricuspid valve

8. Which component of blood helps to fight off diseases?
   a. Red blood cells
   b. White blood cells
   c. Plasma
   d. Platelets

9. Which system consists of a group of organs that work together to transform food and liquids into fuel for the body?
   a. Respiratory system
   b. Immune system
   c. Genitourinary system
   d. Gastrointestinal system

10. During which step, performed by the gastrointestinal system, do chemicals and enzymes break down complex food molecules into smaller molecules?
   a. Digestion
   b. Absorption
   c. Compaction
   d. Ingestion

11. Which accessory organ of the gastrointestinal system is responsible for storing and concentrating bile?
   a. Liver
   b. Pancreas
   c. Stomach
   d. Gallbladder

12. Which type of muscle helps pump blood through the veins and arteries?
   a. Skeletal
   b. Smooth
   c. Intestinal
   d. Cardiac

13. How do neuroglia support neurons?
   a. They provide nutrition to them and help remove waste products.
   b. They provide a framework around them and protect them from the surrounding environment.
   c. They relay messages to them from the brain and from them back to the brain.
   d. They connect them to other surrounding cells.

14. Which nerve system allows the brain to regulate body functions such as heart rate and blood pressure?
   a. Central
   b. Somatic
   c. Autonomic
   d. Afferent

15. Which of the following organs is NOT considered an accessory organ of the male reproductive system?
    a. Testes
    b. Prostate
    c. Vas deferens
    d. Bulbourethral glands

16. How many gametes do the ovaries produce every month?
    a. One million
    b. One
    c. One-half billion
    d. Two

17. In what part of the female reproductive system do sperm fertilize an oocyte?
    a. Ovary
    b. Mammary gland
    c. Vagina
    d. Fallopian tubes

18. What is the largest organ in the human body?
    a. Brain
    b. Large intestine
    c. Skin
    d. Liver

19. Which is a function of the skin?
    a. Temperature regulation
    b. Breathing
    c. Ingestion
    d. Gas exchange

20. Which accessory organ of the integumentary system provides a hard layer of protection over the skin?
    a. Hair
    b. Nails
    c. Sweat glands
    d. Sebaceous glands

21. Which of the following is a distinct characteristic of tissues and glands that are a part of the endocrine system?
    a. They lack a blood supply.
    b. They act quickly in response to stimuli.
    c. They secrete bile.
    d. They are ductless.

22. Which endocrine gland is found at the bottom of the hypothalamus?
    a. Pituitary
    b. Thymus
    c. Thyroid
    d. Pancreas

23. Which endocrine gland regulates the blood sugar levels of the body?
    a. Pineal
    b. Parathyroid
    c. Pancreas
    d. Adrenal

24. Which organ is responsible for filtering waste products out of the bloodstream?
    a. Kidneys
    b. Urinary bladder
    c. Pancreas
    d. Urethra

25. What is the function of the bulbourethral glands?
    a. To produce a fluid that serves as nourishment to the oocyte in the Fallopian tubes
    b. To produce a fluid that lubricates the vaginal canal and neutralizes the residual acidity from urine
    c. To produce a fluid that lubricates the urethra and neutralizes the residual acidity from urine
    d. To produce a fluid that serves as nourishment to the sperm during ejaculation

26. What happens to the urinary bladder as urine enters and is stored until the bladder is emptied?
    a. Blood flow to the organ increases.
    b. It secretes waste into the urine.
    c. Its walls stretch and become thinner.
    d. Its internal pressure increases.

27. Which immune system works in a nonspecific way and does not remember pathogens that it previously fought against?
    a. Innate
    b. Adaptive
    c. Hormonal
    d. B cell

28. How does the adaptive immune system work to fight against previously encountered pathogens?
    a. It sends out all antibodies to inactivate the pathogen.
    b. It sends out target-specific antibodies to inactivate the pathogen.
    c. It uses a mechanical barrier, such as the skin, to protect against pathogens.
    d. It uses a chemical barrier, such as gastric acid, to protect against pathogens.

29. What type of disorder can develop if the immune system is not functioning properly?
    a. Adaptive
    b. Innate
    c. Lymphocytic
    d. Autoimmune

30. How many bones are in the adult human skeletal system?
    a. 206
    b. Three hundred
    c. Twenty-seven
    d. Twenty-six

31. What is the insertion of biceps brachii?
    a. Ulnar notch of the radius
    b. Radial tuberosity
    c. Coronoid process of the ulna
    d. Ulnar head

32. Which structure is superior to the sphenoid bone?
    a. Maxilla
    b. Zygomatic bone
    c. Parietal bones
    d. Occipital bone

33. Which of the following muscles inserts on the anterolateral side of the humerus?
    a. Deltoid
    b. Latissimus dorsi
    c. Brachialis
    d. Biceps brachii

34. Which of the following innervates the flexor digitorum superficialis muscle?
    a. Median nerve
    b. Ulnar nerve
    c. Radial nerve
    d. Axillary nerve

35. Which of the following inserts on the superior side of the patella?
    a. Vastus intermedius muscle
    b. Patellar ligament
    c. Biceps femoris
    d. Quadriceps tendon

Answer Explanations

1. A: There are only two hundred different types of cells in the human body. While there are trillions of cells that make up the human body, only about two hundred different types make up that trillion, each with a specific function.

2. C: Connective tissue is located only on the inside of the body and fills internal spaces. This allows it to protect the organs within the body. Epithelial tissue is found on the outside of the body and as a lining of internal cavities and passageways. Muscle tissue allows for movement of the body. Neural tissue sends information from the brain to the rest of the body through electrical impulses.

3. D: After air enters the nose or mouth, it gets passed on to the sinuses. The sinuses regulate temperature and humidity before passing the air on to the rest of the body. Volume of air can change with varying temperatures and humidity levels, so it is important for the air to be a constant temperature and humidity before being processed by the lungs. The larynx is the voice box of the body, making Choice *A* incorrect. The lungs are responsible for oxygen and carbon dioxide exchange between the air that is breathed in and the blood that is circulating the body, making Choice *B* incorrect. The trachea takes the temperature- and humidity-regulated air from the sinuses to the lungs, making Choice *C* incorrect.

4. D: The bicuspid valve, also called the mitral valve, is on the left side of the heart between the left atrium and left ventricle. It closes after the left ventricle has filled with blood to prevent blood from flowing backward into the atrium. Choice *B* is incorrect because this valve is on the left, not right, side of the heart. Choices *A* and *C* are incorrect because they state the opposite in terms of oxygenation of the blood for the circulation route mentioned. Oxygen-depleted blood from the body enters the right atrium and is pumped into the right ventricle. This blood, which has a high carbon dioxide content then enters pulmonary circulation where it can become re-oxygenated. Oxygen-rich blood from the lungs then flows into the left atrium, passes into the left ventricle, and enters the aorta for systemic circulation.

5. C: The main function of the lungs is to provide oxygen to the blood circulating in the body and to remove carbon dioxide from blood that has already circulated the body. The passageways within the lungs are responsible for this gas exchange between the air and the blood. The nose, Choice *A*, is the first place where air is breathed in. The larynx, Choice *B*, is the voice box of the body. The stomach, Choice *D*, is responsible for getting nutrients out of food and drink that are ingested, not from air.

6. B: The myocardium is the middle layer of the heart wall and contains connective tissue, blood vessels, and nerves. The epicardium, Choice *A*, is the outer layer of the heart wall and is solely made up of a serous membrane without any nerves or blood vessels. The endocardium, Choice *C*, is the inner layer of the heart wall and is made up of a simple squamous epithelium. The sternum, Choice *D*, is the chest bone and protects the heart.

7. A: The mitral valve is also known as the bicuspid valve because it has two leaflets. It is located on the left side of the heart between the atrium and the ventricle. The pulmonary valve, Choice *B*, is located between the right ventricle and the pulmonary artery and has three cusps. The aortic valve, Choice *C*, is located between the left ventricle and the aorta and also has three cusps. The tricuspid valve, Choice *D*, has three leaflets and is located on the right side of the heart between the atrium and the ventricle.

8. B: White blood cells are part of the immune system and help fight off diseases. Red blood cells contain hemoglobin, which carries oxygen through the blood. Plasma is the liquid matrix of the blood. Platelets help with the clotting of the blood.

9. D: The gastrointestinal system consists of the stomach and intestines, which help process food and liquid so that the body can absorb nutrients for fuel. The respiratory system is involved with the exchange of oxygen and carbon dioxide between the air and blood. The immune system helps the body fight against pathogens and diseases. The genitourinary system helps the body to excrete waste.

10. A: During digestion, complex food molecules are broken down into smaller molecules so that nutrients can be isolated and absorbed by the body. Absorption, Choice *B*, is when vitamins, electrolytes, organic molecules, and water are absorbed by the digestive epithelium. Compaction, Choice *C*, occurs when waste products are dehydrated and compacted. Ingestion, Choice *D*, is when food and liquids first enter the body through the mouth.

11. D: The gallbladder is the organ that is responsible for storing and concentrating bile before secreting it into the small intestine. The liver, Choice *A*, is responsible for producing bile. The pancreas, Choice *B*, is responsible for secreting digestive enzymes specific for different types of food. The stomach, Choice *C*, is where digestion occurs.

12. D: Cardiac muscle cells are involuntary and make up the heart muscle, which pumps blood through the veins and arteries. Skeletal muscle, Choice *A*, helps with body movement by pulling on the bones of the skeleton. Smooth muscle, Choice *B*, is an involuntary, nonstriated muscle that is found in the digestive tract and other hollow internal organs, such as the urinary bladder and blood vessels. The intestines, Choice *C*, are made up of smooth muscle cells.

13. B: Neurons are responsible for transferring and processing information between the brain and other parts of the body. Neuroglia are cells that protect delicate neurons by making a frame around them. They also help to maintain a homeostatic environment around the neurons.

14. C: The autonomic nerve system is part of the efferent division of the peripheral nervous system (PNS). It controls involuntary muscles, such as smooth muscle and cardiac muscle, which are responsible for regulating heart rate, blood pressure, and body temperature. The central nervous system, Choice *A*, includes only the brain and the spinal cord. The somatic nervous system, Choice *B*, is also part of the efferent division of the PNS and controls voluntary skeletal muscle contractions, allowing for body movements. The afferent division of the PNS, Choice *D*, relays sensory information within the body.

15. A: The testes are the main reproductive organ of the male reproductive system. They are the gonads; they secrete androgens and produce and store sperm cells. The prostate, vas deferens, and bulbourethral glands are all accessory organs of the male reproductive system. The prostate provides nourishment to sperm, the vas deferens transports sperm to the urethra, and the bulbourethral glands produce lubricating fluid for the urethra.

16. B: The ovaries produce only one mature gamete each month. If it is fertilized, the result is a zygote that develops into an embryo. The male reproductive system produces one-half billion sperm cells each day.

17. D: Once sperm enter the vagina, they travel through the uterus to the fallopian tubes to fertilize a mature oocyte. The ovaries are responsible for producing the mature oocyte. The mammary glands produce nutrient-filled milk to nourish babies after birth.

18. C: The skin is the largest organ of the body, covering every external surface of the body and protecting the body's deeper tissues. The brain performs many complex functions, and the large intestine is part of the gastrointestinal system, but neither of these is largest organ in the body. The liver is the second largest organ of the body, weighing roughly three pounds in the average adult.

19. A: The skin has three major functions: protection, regulation, and sensation. It has a large supply of blood vessels that can dilate to allow heat loss when the body is too hot and constrict in order to retain heat when the body is cold. The organs of respiratory system are responsible for breathing and work together with the circulatory system for gas exchange, and the mouth is responsible for ingestion.

20. B: The nails on a person's hands and feet provide a hard layer of protection over the soft skin underneath. The hair, Choice *A*, helps to protect against heat loss, provides sensation, and filters air that enters the nose. The sweat glands, Choice *C*, help to regulate temperature. The sebaceous glands, Choice *D*, secrete sebum, which protects the skin from water loss and bacterial and fungal infections.

21. D: The tissues and glands of the endocrine system are all ductless. They secrete hormones, not bile, into the blood or interstitial fluid of the human body. The endocrine system has a slow, long-lasting response to stimuli, unlike the nervous system, which produces quick and short-term responses.

22. A: The pituitary gland is a pea-sized gland that is found at the bottom of the hypothalamus. The hormones that it releases regulate growth, blood pressure, and pain relief, among other things. The thymus, Choice *B*, is located in the chest cavity and produces hormones that are important for the development and maintenance of immune responses. The thyroid gland, Choice *C*, is found in the neck and releases hormones responsible for metabolism, growth and development, temperature regulation, and brain development during infancy and childhood. The pancreas, Choice *D*, is located in the abdomen and regulates blood sugar levels.

23. C: The pancreas is responsible for regulating blood sugar levels in the body. The pineal gland regulates melatonin levels, which affects maturation of gametes and reproductive organs, as well as the body's circadian rhythm. The parathyroid gland secretes a hormone that helps the thyroid regulate calcium levels in the body. The adrenal glands help with the body's management of stress.

24. A: The kidneys are the main organs responsible for filtering waste products out of the bloodstream. The kidneys have millions of nephrons, which are tiny filtering units that filter 120 to 150 quarts of blood each day and produce waste, approximately one to two quarts of urine daily. The urinary bladder is responsible for storing urine. The pancreas is responsible for regulating blood sugar levels. The urethra is the passageway through which urine exits the body.

25. C: The bulbourethral glands are part of the male reproductive system. They produce a lubricating fluid for the urethra that also neutralizes the residual acidity left behind by urine. Choice *D* is incorrect because it is the prostate gland and the seminal vesicles, not the bulbourethral glands, that provide additional fluid that nourishes the sperm during ejaculation. In the male genitourinary system, both urine and gametes travel through the urethra to exit the body. The sperm is produced by the testes and then travels through the urethra. Urine is produced by the kidneys, is stored in the urinary bladder, and then exits the body through the urethra. In females, the urethra is solely used for urine to exit the body. Gametes exit the body from the uterus and through the vagina. Females do not have bulbourethral glands, so Choices *A* and *B* are incorrect.

26. C: The urinary bladder is a hollow, elastic muscular organ. As it fills with urine, the walls stretch without breaking—due to their elasticity—and become thinner. When the urine is emptied, the bladder returns to its original size. The urinary bladder does not secrete any fluids into the urine; it is a storage organ for urine. Pressure inside the urinary bladder does not increase as it is filled because the organ grows larger while filling.

27. A: The innate immune system works based on pattern recognition of similar pathogens that have already been encountered. It does not remember specific pathogens or provide an individually-specific response. The responses it provides are short term and do not work toward long-lasting immunity for the body. The adaptive immune system creates a memory of each specific pathogen that has been encountered and provides a pathogen-specific response. This works toward the long-term immunity of the body. Hormones are secreted by the endocrine system in response to stimuli. B cells are lymphocytes that work to provide immunity as part of the adaptive immune system.

28. B: The adaptive immune system provides target-specific antibodies to fight against individual pathogens that are encountered. It does not send out a broad range of antibodies because it has memory of the previously encountered pathogens. Mechanical and chemical barriers are part of the innate immune system and do not provide target-specific immunity.

29. D: If the immune system is not functioning properly, it may begin to attack its own healthy cells, which can result in an autoimmune disorder, such as celiac disease, type I diabetes, or rheumatoid arthritis. The adaptive and innate immune systems are the two parts of the body's immune system that need to be working properly to protect the body from pathogens. Lymphocytes are specialized cells that help the adaptive immune system provide target-specific responses to pathogens.

30. A: There are 206 bones in the adult human body. Human babies are born with three hundred bones. As they grow, bones fuse together and the body is left with 206 individual bones. There are twenty-seven bones in one human hand and twenty-six bones in one human foot.

31. B: Biceps brachii inserts at the radial tuberosity, the rough spot located on the medial side of the radius, inferior to the neck of the radius. The ulnar notch of the radius is the distal indentation that accommodates the head of the ulna. The coronoid process of the ulna is an insertion for the brachialis muscle, not biceps brachii.

32. C: The sphenoid bone is one of the bones of the neurocranium and is part of the orbit. The parietal bone is superior and posterior to the sphenoid bone. The maxilla is the nonmotile, upper jaw. The zygomatic bone is part of the facial skeleton and is anterior and lateral to the sphenoid bone. The occipital bone is another bone in the neurocranium, but it is located inferior and posterior to the sphenoid bone.

33. A: The deltoid muscle inserts on the anterolateral side of the humerus. Latissimus dorsi inserts on the humerus, but on the intertubercular groove, found on the anteromedial side of the humerus proximal to the head. The brachialis instead originates on the anterior side of the humerus and inserts on the ulna. Biceps brachii crosses the humerus but does not insert or originate on it.

34. A: The flexor digitorum superficialis, which flexes the wrist and fingers, is innervated by the median nerve, which is supplied by the lateral cord and medial cord. The ulnar nerve is located medially in the forearm, stemming from the medial cord. The radial nerve primarily innervates the posterior muscles of the upper arm and forearm including the triceps. The axillary nerve is located in the upper arm and innervates the deltoid and teres minor in the shoulder.

35. D: The quadriceps tendon inserts on the superior side of the patella, and originates from the four muscles making up the quadriceps, including the vastus intermedius muscle. The patellar ligament is inferior to the patella, connecting it to the tibia. The biceps femoris is a posterior muscle in the thigh which serves to flex the knee.

Physics

Nature of Motion

Cultures have been studying the movement of objects since ancient times. These studies have been prompted by curiosity and sometimes by necessity. On Earth, items move according to guidelines and have motion that is fairly predictable. To understand why an object moves along its path, it is important to understand what role forces have on influencing its movements. The term *force* describes an outside influence on an object. Force does not have to refer to something imparted by another object. Forces can act upon objects by touching them with a push or a pull, by friction, or without touch like a magnetic force or even gravity. Forces can affect the motion of an object.

To study an object's motion, it must be located and described. When locating an object's position, it can help to pinpoint its location relative to another known object. Comparing an object with respect to a known object is referred to as *establishing a frame of reference*. If the placement of one object is known, it is easier to locate another object with respect to the position of the original object.

Motion can be described by following specific guidelines called *kinematics*. Kinematics use mechanics to describe motion without regard to the forces that are causing such motions. Specific equations can be used when describing motions; these equations use time as a frame of reference. The equations are based on the change of an object's position (represented by x), over a change in time (represented by Δt). This describes an object's velocity, which is measured in meters/second (m/s) and described by the following equation:

$$v = \frac{\Delta x}{\Delta t} = \frac{x_f - x_i}{\Delta t}$$

Velocity is a vector quantity, meaning it measures the magnitude (how much) and the direction that the object is moving. Both of these components are essential to understanding and predicting the motion of objects. The scientist Isaac Newton did extensive studies on the motion of objects on Earth and came up with three primary laws to describe motion:

Law 1: An object in motion tends to stay in motion unless acted upon by an outside force. An object at rest tends to stay at rest unless acted upon by an outside force (also known as the *law of inertia*).

For example, if a book is placed on a table, it will stay there until it is moved by an outside force.

Law 2: The force acting upon an object is equal to the object's mass multiplied by its acceleration (also known as F = ma).

For example, the amount of force acting on a bug being swatted by a flyswatter can be calculated if the mass of the flyswatter and its acceleration are known. If the mass of the flyswatter is 0.3 kg and the acceleration of its swing is 2.0 m/s^2, the force of its swing can be calculated as follows:

$$m = 0.3\, kg$$
$$a = 2.0\, m/s^2$$
$$F = m \times a$$
$$F = (0.3) \times (2.0)$$
$$F = 0.6\, N$$

Law 3: For every action, there is an equal and opposite reaction.

For example, when a person claps their hands together, the right hand feels the same force as the left hand, as the force is equal and opposite.

Another example is if a car and a truck run head-on into each other, the force experienced by the truck is equal and opposite to the force experienced by the car, regardless of their respective masses or velocities. The ability to withstand this amount of force is what varies between the vehicles and creates a difference in the amount of damage sustained.

Newton used these laws to describe motion and derive additional equations for motion that could predict the position, velocity, acceleration, or time for objects in motion in one and two dimensions. Since all of Newton's work was done on Earth, he primarily used Earth's gravity and the behavior of falling objects to design experiments and studies in free fall (an object subject to Earth's gravity while in flight). On Earth, the acceleration due to the force of gravity is measured at 9.8 meters per second^2 (m/s^2). This value is the same for anything on the Earth or within Earth's atmosphere.

Acceleration

Acceleration is the change in velocity over the change in time. It is given by the following equation:

$$a = \frac{\Delta v}{\Delta t} = \frac{v_f - v_i}{\Delta t}$$

Since velocity is the change in position (displacement) over a change in time, it is necessary for calculating an acceleration. Both of these are vector quantities, meaning they have magnitude and direction (or some amount in some direction). Acceleration is measured in units of distance over time^2 (meters/second^2 or m/s^2 in metric units).

For example, what is the acceleration of a vehicle that has an initial velocity of 35 m/s and a final velocity of 10 m/s over 5.0 s?

Using the givens and the equation:

$$a = \frac{\Delta v}{\Delta t} = \frac{v_f - v_i}{\Delta t}$$

V_f = 10 m/s

V_i = 35 m/s

Δt = 5.0 s

$$a = \frac{10 - 35}{5.0} = \frac{-25}{5.0} = -5.0 \, m/s^2$$

The vehicle is decelerating at −5.0 m/s^2.

If an object is moving with a constant velocity, its velocity does not change over time. Therefore, it has no (or 0) acceleration.

It is common to misuse vector terms in spoken language. For example, people frequently use the term "speed" in situations where the correct term would be "velocity." However, the difference between velocity and speed is not just that velocity must have a direction component with it. Average velocity and average speed actually are looking at two different distances as well. Average speed is calculated simply by dividing the total distance covered by the time it took to travel that distance. If someone runs four miles along a straight road north and then makes a 90-degree turn to the right and runs another three miles down that straight road east (such that the runner's route of seven miles makes up two sides of a rectangle) in seventy minutes, the runner's average speed was 6 miles per hour (one mile covered every ten minutes). Using the same course, the runner's average velocity would be about 4.29 miles per hour northeast.

Why is the magnitude less in the case of velocity? Velocity measures the change in position, or **displacement**, which is the shortest line between the starting point and ending point. Even if the path between these two points is serpentine or meanders all over the place racking up a great distance, the displacement is still just the shortest straight path between the change in the position of the object. In the case of the runner, the "distance" used to calculate velocity (the displacement) is the hypotenuse of the triangle that would connect the two side lengths at right angles to one another. Using basic trigonometric ratios, we know this distance is 5 miles (since the lengths of the other two legs are 3 miles and 4 miles and the Pythagorean Theorem says that $a^2 + b^2 = c^2$). Therefore, although the distance the runner covered was seven miles, their displacement was only five miles. Average velocity is thus calculated by taking the total time (70 minutes) and dividing it by the displacement (5 miles northeast). Therefore, to calculate average velocity of the runner, 70 minutes is divided by 5 miles, so each mile of displacement to the northeast was covered in 14 minutes. To find this rate in miles per hour, 60 minutes is divided by 14, to get 4.29 miles per hour northeast.

Another misconception is if something has a negative acceleration, it must be slowing down. If the change in position of the moving object is in a negative direction, it could have a negative velocity. If the acceleration is in the same direction as this negative velocity, it would be increasing the velocity in the negative direction, thus resulting in the object actually increasing in velocity.

For example, if west is designated to be a negative direction, a car increasing in speed to the west would have a negative velocity. Since it is increasing in speed, it would be accelerating in the negative direction, resulting in a negative acceleration.

Another common misconception is if a person is running around an oval track at a constant velocity, they would have no (or 0) acceleration because there is no change in the runner's velocity. This idea is incorrect because the person is changing direction the entire time they are running around the track, so there would be a change in their velocity. Therefore, the runner would have an acceleration.

One final point regarding acceleration is that it can result from the force a rotating body exerts toward its center. For planets and other massive bodies, it is called *gravity*. This type of acceleration can also be utilized to separate substances, as in a centrifuge.

Projectile Motion

When objects are launched or thrown into the air, they exhibit what is called **projectile motion**. This motion takes a parabolic (or arced) path as the object rises and/or falls with the effect of gravity. In sports, if a ball is thrown across a field, it will follow a path of projectile motion. Whatever angle the object leaves the horizon is the same angle with which it will return to the horizon. The height the object achieves is referred to as the **y-component**, and the distance along the horizon the object travels is referred to as the **x-component**. To maximize the horizontal distance an object travels, it should be launched at a 45-degree angle relative to the horizon. The following shows the range, or x-distance, an object can travel when launched at various angles:

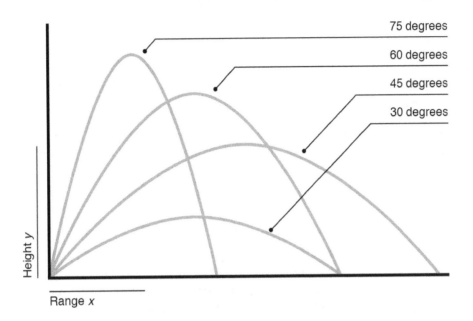

If something is traveling through the air without an internal source of power or any extra external forces acting upon it, it will follow these paths. All projectiles experience the effects of gravity while on Earth; therefore, they will experience a constant acceleration of 9.8 m/s^2 in a downward direction. While on its path, a projectile will have both a horizontal and vertical component to its motion and velocity. At the launch, the object has both vertical and horizontal velocity. As the object increases in height, the y-component of its velocity will diminish until the very peak of the object's path. At the peak, the y-component of the velocity is zero. Since the object still has a horizontal, or x-component, to its velocity, it would continue its motion. There is also a constant acceleration of 9.8 m/s^2 acting in the downward direction on the object the entire time, so at the peak of the object's height, the velocity would then switch from zero to being pulled down with the acceleration. The entire path of the object takes a specific amount of time, based on the initial launch angle and velocity. The time and distance traveled can be calculated using the kinematic equations of motion. The time it takes the object to reach its maximum height is exactly half of the time for the object's entire flight.

Similar motion is exhibited if an object is thrown from atop a building, bridge, cliff, etc. Since it would be starting at its maximum height, the motion of the object would be comparable to the second half of the path in the above diagram.

Newton's Laws of Motion

Newton's laws of motion describe the relationship between an object and the forces acting upon that object, and its movement responding to those forces. Although previously explained, it's helpful to again summarize **Newton's three laws of motion**:

Law of Inertia: An object at rest stays at rest and an object in motion stays in motion unless otherwise acted upon by an outside force. For example, gravity is an outside force that will affect the speed and direction of a ball; when we throw a ball, the ball will eventually decrease in speed and fall to the ground because of the outside force of gravity. However, if the ball were kicked in space where there is no gravity, the ball would go the same speed and direction forever unless it hits another object in space or falls into another gravity field.

F=ma: This law states that the heavier an object, the more force required to move it. This force has to do with acceleration. For example, if you use the same amount of force to push both a golf cart and an eighteen-wheeler, the golf cart will have more acceleration than the truck because the eighteen-wheeler weighs more than the golf cart.

Law of reactions: This law states that for every action, there is an opposite and equal reaction. For example, if you are jumping on a trampoline, you are experiencing Newton's third law of motion. When a book is slammed down on a table, the table pushes back up on the book with a force of equal magnitude but in the opposite direction.

Friction

As previously stated with Newton's laws, forces act upon objects on the Earth. If an object is resting on a surface, the effect of gravity acting upon its mass produces a force referred to as *weight*. This weight touches the surface it is resting on, and the surface produces a normal force perpendicular to this surface. If an outside force acts upon this object, its movement will be resisted by the surfaces rubbing on each other.

Friction is the term used to describe the force that opposes motion, or the force experienced when two surfaces interact with each other. Every surface has a specific amount with which it resists motion, called a *coefficient of friction*. The coefficient of friction is a proportion calculated from the force of friction divided by the normal force (force produced perpendicular to a surface).

$$\mu_s = \frac{F_s}{F_N}$$

There are different types of friction between surfaces. If something is at rest, it has a static (non-moving) friction. It requires an outside force to begin its movement. The coefficient of static friction for that material multiplied by the normal force would need to be greater than the force of static friction to get the object moving. Therefore, the force required to move an object must be greater than the force of static friction:

$$F_s \leq \mu_s \times F_N$$

Once the object is in motion, the force required to maintain this movement only needs to be equivalent to the value of the force of kinetic (moving) friction. To calculate the force of kinetic friction, simply multiply the coefficient of kinetic friction for that surface by the normal force:

$$F_k = \mu_k \times F_N$$

The force required to start an object in motion is larger than the force required to continue its motion once it has begun:

$$F_s \geq F_k$$

Friction not only occurs between solid surfaces; it also occurs in air and liquids. In air, it is called *air resistance*, or drag, and in water, it is called *viscosity*.

For example, what would the coefficient of static friction be if a 5.0 N force was applied to push a 20 kg crate, from rest, across a flat floor?

First, the normal force could be found to counter the force from the weight of the object, which would be the mass multiplied by gravity:

$$F_N = mass \times gravity$$

$$F_N = 20 \ kg \times 9.8 \ \frac{m}{s^2}$$

$$F_N = 196 \ N$$

Next, the coefficient of static friction could be found by dividing the frictional force by the normal force:

$$\mu_s = \frac{F_s}{F_N}$$

$$\mu_s = \frac{5.0 \ N}{196 \ N}$$

$$\mu_s = 0.03$$

Since it is a coefficient, the units cancel out, so the solution is unitless. The coefficient of static friction should also be less than 1.0.

Rotation

An object moving on a circular path has momentum (a measurement of an object's mass and velocity in a direction); for circular motion, it is called **angular momentum**, and this value is determined by rotational inertia, rotational velocity, and the distance of the mass from the axis of rotation, or the center of rotation.

If objects are exhibiting circular motion, they are demonstrating the conservation of angular momentum. The angular momentum of a system is always constant, regardless of the placement of the mass. As stated above, the rotational inertia of an object can be affected by how far the mass of the object is placed with respect to the center of rotation (*axis of rotation*). A larger distance between the mass and the center of rotation means a slower rotational velocity. Reversely, if a mass is closer to the center of rotation, the rotational velocity increases. A change in the placement of the mass affects the value of the rotational velocity, thus conserving the angular momentum. This is true as long as no external forces act upon the system.

For example, if an ice skater is spinning on one ice skate and extends their arms out (or increases the distance between the mass and the center of rotation), a slower rotational velocity is created. When the skater brings the arms in close to the body (or lessens the distance between the mass and the center of rotation), their rotational velocity increases, and he or she spins much faster. Some skaters extend their arms straight up above their head, which causes the axis of rotation to extend, thus removing any distance between the mass and the center of rotation and maximizing the rotational velocity.

Consider another example. If a person is selecting a horse on a merry-go-round, the placement of their selection can affect their ride experience. All the horses are traveling with the same rotational speed, but to travel along the same plane as the merry-go-round, a horse closer to the outside will have a greater linear speed due to being farther away from the axis of rotation. Another way to think of this is that an outside horse must cover more distance than a horse near the inside to keep up with the rotational speed of the merry-go-round platform. Based on this information, thrill seekers should always select an outer horse to experience a greater linear speed.

Uniform Circular Motion

When an object exhibits circular motion, its motion is centered around an axis. An **axis** is an invisible line on which an object can rotate. This type of motion is most easily observed on a toy top. There is actually a point (or rod) through the center of the top on which the top can be observed to be spinning. This is also called the axis. An axis is the location about which the mass of an object or system would rotate if free to spin.

In the instance of utilizing a lever to lift an object, it can be helpful to calculate the amount of force needed at a specific distance, applied perpendicular to the axis of motion, to calculate the torque, or circular force, necessary to move something. This is also employed when using a wrench to loosen a bolt. The equation for calculating the force in a circular direction, or perpendicular to an axis, is as follows:

$$Torque = F_\perp \times distance\ of\ lever\ arm\ from\ the\ axis\ of\ rotation$$

$$\tau = F_\perp \times d$$

For example, what torque would result from a 20 N force being applied to a lever 5 meters from its axis of rotation?

$$\tau = 20\,N \times 5\,m$$

$$\tau = 100\,N \times m$$

The amount of torque would be 100 N×m. The units would be Newton meters because it is a force applied at a distance away from the axis of rotation.

When objects move in a circle by spinning on their own axis, or because they are tethered around a central point (also considered an axis), they exhibit circular motion. Circular motion is similar in many ways to linear (straight line) motion; however, there are some additional facts to note. When an object spins or rotates on or around an axis, a force that feels like it is pushing out from the center of the circle is created. The force is actually pulling into the center of the circle. A reactionary force is what is creating the feeling of pushing out. The inward force is the real force, and this is called **centripetal force**. The outward, or reactionary, force is called **centrifugal force**. The reactionary force is not the real force; it just feels like it is there. This can also be referred to as a **fictional force**. The true force is the one pulling inward, or the centripetal force. The terms *centripetal* and *centrifugal* are often mistakenly interchanged.

For example, the method a traditional-style washing machine uses to spin a load of clothes to expunge the water from the load is to spin the machine barrel in a circle at a high rate of speed. During this spinning, the centripetal force is pulling in toward the center of the circle. At the same time, the reactionary force to the centripetal force is pressing the clothes up against the outer sides of the barrel, which expels the water out of the small holes that line the outer wall of the barrel.

Kinetic Energy and Potential Energy

There are two main types of energy. The first type is called **potential energy** (or gravitational potential energy), and it is stored energy, or energy due to an object's height from the ground.

The second type is called **kinetic energy**. Kinetic energy is the energy of motion. If an object is moving, it will have some amount of kinetic energy.

For example, if a roller-coaster car is sitting on the track at the top of a hill, it would have all potential energy and no kinetic energy. As the roller coaster travels down the hill, the energy converts from potential energy into kinetic energy. At the bottom of the hill, where the car is traveling the fastest, it would have all kinetic energy and no potential energy.

Another measure of energy is the total mechanical energy in a system. This is the sum (or total) of the potential energy plus the kinetic energy of the system. The total mechanical energy in a system is always conserved. The amounts of the potential energy and kinetic energy in a system can vary, but the total mechanical energy in a situation would remain the same.

The equation for the mechanical energy in a system is as follows:

$$ME = PE + KE$$

$$(Mechanical\ Energy\ =\ Potential\ Energy\ +\ Kinetic\ Energy)$$

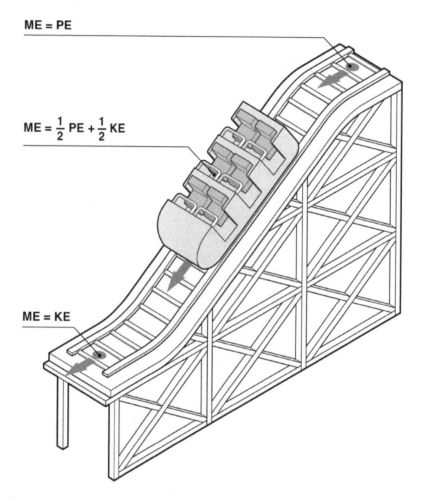

Energy can transfer or change forms, but it cannot be created or destroyed. This transfer can take place through waves (including light waves and sound waves), heat, impact, etc.

There is a fundamental law of thermodynamics (the study of heat and movement) called **conservation of energy**. This law states that energy cannot be created or destroyed, but rather energy is transferred to different forms involved in a process. For instance, a car pushed beginning at one end of a street will not continue down that street forever; it will gradually come to a stop some distance away from where it was originally pushed. This does not mean the energy has disappeared or has been exhausted; it means the energy has been transferred to different mediums surrounding the car. Some of the energy is dissipated by the frictional force from the road on the tires, the air resistance from the movement of the car, the sound from the tires on the road, and the force of gravity pulling on the car. Each value can be calculated in a number of ways, including measuring the sound waves from the tires, the temperature change in the tires, the distance moved by the car from start to finish, etc. It is important to understand that many processes factor into such a small situation, but all situations follow the conservation of energy.

Just like the earlier example, the roller coaster at the top of a hill has a measurable amount of potential energy; when it rolls down the hill, it converts most of that energy into kinetic energy. There are still additional factors such as friction and air resistance working on the coaster and dissipating some of the energy, but energy transfers in every situation.

There are six basic machines that utilize the transfer of energy to the advantage of the user. These machines function based on an amount of energy input from the user and accomplish a task by distributing the energy for a common purpose. These machines are called *simple machines* and include the lever, pulley, wedge, inclined plane, screw, and wheel and axle.

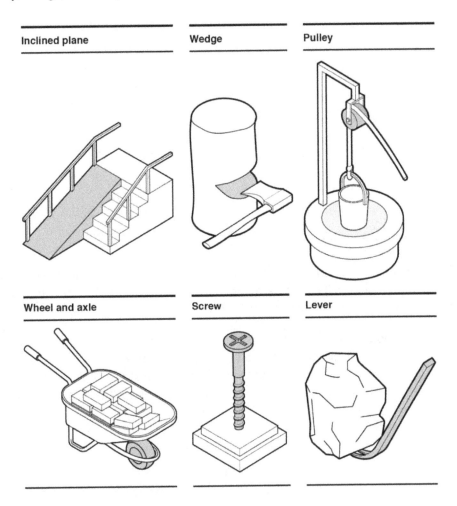

The use of simple machines can help by requiring less force to perform a task with the same result. This is referred to as a **mechanical advantage**.

For example, if a father is trying to lift his child into the air with his arms to pick an apple from a tree, it would require less force to place the child on one end of a teeter totter and push the other end of the teeter totter down to elevate the child to the same height to pick the apple. In this example, the teeter totter is a lever.

Linear Momentum and Impulse

The motion of an object can be expressed as momentum. This is a calculation of an object's mass times its velocity. **Momentum** can be described as the amount an object will continue moving along its current course. Momentum in a straight line is called *linear momentum*. Just as energy can be transferred and conserved, so can momentum.

Momentum is denoted by the letter *p* and calculated by multiplying an object's mass by its velocity.

$$p = m \times v$$

For example, if a car and a truck are moving at the same velocity (25 meters per second) down a highway, they will not have the same momentum because they do not have the same mass. The mass of the truck (3500 kg) is greater than that of the car (1000 kg); therefore, the truck will have more momentum. In a head-on collision, the truck's momentum is greater than the car's, and the truck will cause more damage to the car than the car will to the truck. The equations to compare the momentum of the car and the truck are as follows:

$$p_{truck} = mass_{truck} \times velocity_{truck} \qquad p_{car} = mass_{car} \times velocity_{car}$$

$$p_{truck} = 3500 \; kg \times 25 \; m/s \qquad p_{car} = 1000 \; kg \times 25 \; m/s$$

$$p_{truck} = 87{,}500 \; N \qquad p_{car} = 25{,}000 \; N$$

The momentum of the truck is greater than that of the car.

The amount of force during a length of time creates an impulse. This means if a force acts on an object during a given amount of time, it will have a determined impulse. However, if the length of time can be extended, the force will be less due to the conservation of momentum.

For a car crash, the total momentum of each car before the collision would need to equal the total momentum of the cars after the collision. There are two main types of collisions: elastic and inelastic. For the example with a car crash, in an elastic collision, the cars would be separate before the collision, and they would remain separated after the collision. In the case of an inelastic collision, the cars would be separate before the collision, but they would be stuck together after the collision. The only difference would be in the way the momentum is calculated.

For elastic collisions:

$$total \; momentum_{before} = total \; momentum_{after}$$

$$(mass_{car \; 1} \times velocity_{car \; 1}) + (mass_{car \; 2} \times velocity_{car \; 2})$$
$$= (mass_{car \; 1} + mass_{car \; 2}) \times velocity_{car \; 1 \; \& \; car \; 2}$$

The damage from an impact can be lessened by extending the time of the actual impact. This is called the *measure of the impulse of a collision*. It can be calculated by multiplying the change in momentum by the amount of time involved in the impact.

$$I = change \; in \; momentum \times time$$

$$I = \Delta p \times time$$

212

If the time is extended, the force (or change in momentum) is decreased. Conversely, if the time is shortened, the force (or change in momentum) is increased. For example, when catching a fast baseball, it helps soften the blow of the ball to follow through, or cradle the catch. This technique is simply extending the time of the application of the force of the ball so the impact of the ball does not hurt the hand.

For example, if martial arts experts want to break a board by executing a chop from their hands, they need to exert a force on a small point on the board, extremely quickly. If they slow down the time of the impact from the force of their hands, they will probably injure their striking hand and not break the board.

Often, law enforcement officials will use rubber bullets instead of regular bullets to apprehend a criminal. The benefit of the rubber bullet is that the elastic material of the bullet bounces off the target but hits the target with nearly the same momentum as a regular bullet. Since the length of time the rubber bullet is in contact with the target is decreased, the amount of force from the bullet is increased. This method can knock a subject off their feet by the large force and the short time of the impact without causing any lasting harm to the individual. The difference in the types of collisions is noted through the rubber bullet bouncing off the individual, so both the bullet and the subject are separate before the collision and separate after the collision. With a regular bullet, the bullet and subject are separate before the collision, but a regular bullet would most likely not be separated by the subject after the collision.

Universal Gravitation

Every object in the universe that has mass causes an attractive force to every other object in the universe. The amount of attractive force depends on the masses of the two objects in question and the distance that separates the objects. This is called the **law of universal gravitation** and is represented by the following equation:

$$F = G\frac{m_1 m_2}{r^2}$$

In this equation, the force, F, between two objects, m_1 and m_2, is indirectly proportional to the square of the distance separating the two objects. A general gravitational constant G ($6.67 \times 10^{-11}\ \frac{N \cdot m^2}{kg^2}$) is multiplied by the equation. This constant is quite small, so for the force between two objects to be noticeable, they must have sizable masses.

To better understand this on a large scale, a prime representation could be viewed by satellites (planets) in the solar system and the effect they have on each other. All bodies in the universe have an attractive force between them. This is closely seen by the relationship between the Earth and the moon. The Earth and the moon both have a gravitational attraction that affects each other. The moon is smaller in mass than the Earth; therefore, it will not have as big of an influence as the Earth has on it. The attractive force from the moon is observed by the systematic push and pull on the water on the face of the Earth by the rotations the moon makes around the Earth. The tides in oceans and lakes are caused by the moon's gravitational effect on the Earth. Since the moon and the Earth have an attractive force between them, the moon pulls on the side of the Earth closest to the moon, causing the waters to swell (high tide) on that side and leave the ends 90 degrees away from the moon, causing a low tide there. The water on the side of the Earth farthest from the moon experiences the least amount of gravitational attraction so it collects on that side in a high tide.

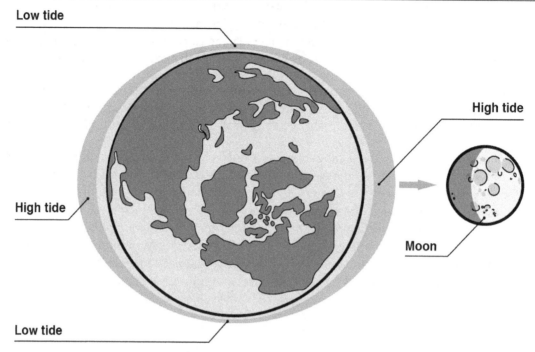

The universal law of gravitation is taken primarily from the works of Johannes Kepler and his laws of planetary motion. These include the fact that the paths of the orbits of the planets are not perfect circles, but ellipses, around the sun. The area swept out between the planet and the sun is equal at every point in the orbit due to fluctuation in speed at different distances. Finally, the period (T) of a planet's motion squared is inversely proportional to the distance (r) between that planet and the sun cubed.

$$\frac{T^2}{r^3}$$

Sir Isaac Newton used this third law and applied it to the idea of forces and their effects on objects. The effect of the gravitational forces of the moon on the Earth are noted in the tides, and the effect of the forces of the Earth on the moon are noted in the fact that the moon is caught in an orbit around the earth. Since the moon is traveling at a velocity tangent to its orbit around the Earth and the Earth keeps attracting it in, the moon does not escape and does not crash into the Earth. The moon will continue this course due to the attractive gravitational force between the Earth and the moon. Albert Einstein later applied Newton's adaptation of Kepler's laws. Einstein was able to develop a more advanced theory, which could explain the motions of all the planets and even be applied beyond the solar system. These theories have also been beneficial for predicting behaviors of other objects in the Earth's atmosphere, such as shuttles and astronauts.

Waves and Sound

Mechanical waves are a type of wave that pass through a medium (solid, liquid, or gas). There are two basic types of mechanical waves: longitudinal and transverse.

A *longitudinal wave* has motion that is parallel to the direction of the wave's travel. It can best be shown by compressing one side of a tethered spring and then releasing that end. The movement travels in a bunching and then unbunching motion, across the length of the spring and back until the energy is dissipated through noise and heat.

A *transverse wave* has motion that is perpendicular to the direction of the wave's travel. The particles on a transverse wave do not move across the length of the wave but oscillate up and down to create the peaks and troughs observed on this type of wave.

A wave with a mix of both longitudinal and transverse motion can be seen through the motion of a wave on the ocean, with peaks and troughs, oscillating particles up and down.

Mechanical waves can carry energy, sound, and light. Mechanical waves need a medium through which transport can take place. However, an electromagnetic wave can transmit energy without a medium, or in a vacuum.

Sound travels in waves and is the movement of vibrations through a medium. It can travel through air (gas), land, water, etc. For example, the noise a human hears in the air is the vibration of the waves as they reach the ear. The human brain translates the different frequencies (pitches) and intensities of the vibrations to determine what created the noise.

A **tuning fork** has a predetermined frequency because of the size (length and thickness) of its tines. When struck, it allows vibrations between the two tines to move the air at a specific rate. This creates a specific tone (or note) for that size of tuning fork. The number of vibrations over time is also steady for that tuning fork and can be matched with a frequency (the number of occurrences over time). All sounds heard by the human ear are categorized by using frequency and measured in hertz (the number of cycles per second).

The intensity (or loudness) of sound is measured on the Bel scale. This scale is a ratio of one sound's intensity with respect to a standard value. It is a logarithmic scale, meaning it is measured by factors of ten. But the value that is 1/10 of this value, the decibel, is the measurement used more commonly for the intensity of pitches heard by the human ear.

The **Doppler effect** applies to situations with both light and sound waves. The premise of the Doppler effect is that, based on the relative position or movement of a source and an observer, waves can seem shorter or longer than they are. When the Doppler effect is experienced with sound, it warps the noise being heard by the observer by making the pitch or frequency seem shorter or higher as the source is approaching and then longer or lower as the source is getting farther away. The frequency and pitch of the source never actually change, but the sound in respect to the observer's position makes it seem like the sound has changed. This effect can be observed when an emergency siren passes by an observer on the road. The siren sounds much higher in pitch as it approaches the observer and then lower after it passes and is getting farther away.

The Doppler effect also applies to situations involving light waves. An observer in space would see light approaching as being shorter wavelengths than it was, causing it to appear blue. When the light wave is getting farther away, the light would look red due to the apparent elongation of the wavelength. This is called the *red-blue shift*.

A recent addition to the study of waves is the gravitational wave. Its existence has been proven and verified, yet the details surrounding its capabilities are still under inquiry. Further understanding of gravitational waves could help scientists understand the beginnings of the universe and how the existence of the solar system is possible. This understanding could also include the future exploration of the universe.

Light

The movement of light is described like the movement of waves. Light travels with a wave front and has an amplitude (a height measured from the neutral), a cycle or wavelength, a period, and energy. Light travels at approximately 3.00×10^8 m/s and is faster than anything created by humans.

Light is commonly referred to by its measured wavelengths, or the length for it to complete one cycle. Types of light with the longest wavelengths include radio, TV, micro, and infrared waves. The next set of wavelengths are detectable by the human eye and make up the visible spectrum. The visible spectrum has wavelengths of 10^{-7} m, and the colors seen are red, orange, yellow, green, blue, indigo, and violet. Beyond the visible spectrum are even shorter wavelengths (also called the *electromagnetic spectrum*) containing ultraviolet light, x-rays, and gamma rays. The wavelengths outside of the visible light range can be harmful to humans if they are directly exposed, especially for long periods of time.

When a wave crosses a boundary or travels from one medium to another, certain actions take place. If the wave travels through one medium into another, it experiences *refraction*, which is the bending of the wave from one medium's density to another, altering the speed of the wave.

For example, a side view of a pencil in half a glass of water appears as though it is bent at the water level. What the viewer is seeing is the refraction of light waves traveling from the air into the water. Since the wave speed is slowed in water, the change makes the pencil appear bent.

When a wave hits a medium that it cannot pass through, it is bounced back in an action called *reflection*. For example, when light waves hit a mirror, they are reflected, or bounced off, the back of the mirror. This can cause it to seem like there is more light in the room due to the doubling back of the initial wave. This is also how people can see their reflection in a mirror.

When a wave travels through a slit or around an obstacle, it is known as *diffraction*. A light wave will bend around an obstacle or through a slit and cause a diffraction pattern. When the waves bend around an obstacle, it causes the addition of waves and the spreading of light on the other side of the opening.

Optics

The dispersion of light describes the splitting of a single wave by refracting its components into separate parts. For example, if a wave of white light is sent through a dispersion prism, the light wave appears as its separate rainbow-colored components due to each colored wavelength being refracted in the prism.

Different things occur when wavelengths of light hit boundaries. Objects can absorb certain wavelengths of light and reflect others, depending on the boundaries. This becomes important when an object appears to be a certain color. The color of the object is not actually within the makeup of that object, but by what wavelengths are being transmitted by that object. For example, if a table appears to be red, that means the table is absorbing all wavelengths of visible light except those of the red wavelength. The table is reflecting, or transmitting, the wavelengths associated with red back to the human eye, and therefore, the table appears red.

Interference describes when an object affects the path of a wave or another wave interacts with that wave. Waves interacting with each other can result in either constructive interference or destructive interference based on their positions. For constructive interference, the waves are in sync and combine to reinforce each other. In the case of deconstructive interference, the waves are out of sync and reduce the effect of each other to some degree. In scattering, the boundary can change the direction or energy of a wave, thus altering the entire wave. Polarization changes the oscillations of a wave and can alter its appearance in light waves. For example, polarized sunglasses take away the "glare" from sunlight by altering the oscillation pattern observed by the wearer.

When a wave hits a boundary and is completely reflected back or cannot escape from one medium to another, it is called *total internal reflection*. This effect can be seen in a diamond with a brilliant cut. The angle cut on the sides of the diamond causes the light hitting the diamond to be completely reflected back inside the gem and makes it appear brighter and more colorful than a diamond with different angles cut into its surface.

When reflecting light, a mirror can be used to observe a virtual (not real) image. A plane mirror is a piece of glass with a coating in the background to create a reflective surface. An image is what the human eye sees when light is reflected off the mirror in an unmagnified manner. If a curved mirror is used for reflection, the image seen will not be a true reflection, but will either be magnified or made to appear smaller than its actual size. Curved mirrors can also make an object appear closer or farther away than its actual distance from the mirror.

Lenses can be used to refract or bend light to form images. Examples of lenses are human eye, microscopes, and telescopes. The human eye interprets the refraction of light into images that humans understand to be actual size. When objects are too small to be observed by the unaided human eye, microscopes allow the objects to be enlarged enough to be seen. Telescopes allow objects that are too far away to be seen by the unaided eye to be viewed. Prisms are pieces of glass that can have a wavelength of light enter one side and appear to be broken down into its component wavelengths on the other side, due to the slowing of certain wavelengths within the prism, more than other wavelengths.

Atomic Structure

Bohr's model of the atom is the one most commonly used model in science today. It was proposed by physicist Niels Bohr and caused some controversy with its configuration of the electrons and their location within the atom. The Bohr model of the atom consists of the nucleus, or core, which is made up of positively-charged protons and neutrally-charged neutrons. The neutrons are theorized to be in the nucleus with the protons. This pairing of protons and neutrons provides a "balance" at the center of the atom. The nucleus of the atom consists of more than 99 percent of the mass of an atom. Surrounding the nucleus are orbitals containing negatively-charged electrons. The entire structure of an atom is too small to be seen with the unaided eye, which has contributed to the differing ideas about its structure. Most research has been focused around recording the reactions of the atom or the energy emitted from the electrons to test any theories about its structure.

Each atom has an atomic number that is assigned by the number of protons within the atom's nucleus. If a substance is made up of atoms that all have the same atomic number, it is called an *element*. Elements are organized by their atomic number and grouped by similar properties in a chart called the **Periodic Table**.

Bohr's Model

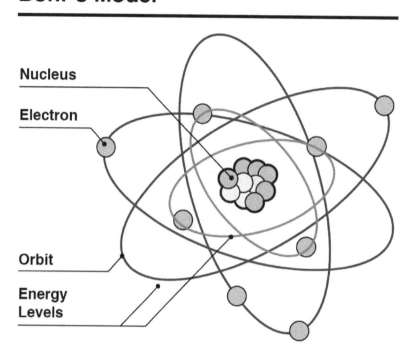

Adding the total number of protons to the total number of neutrons in an atom provides the *mass number*. Most nuclei of atoms are electronically neutral, and all atoms of one type have the same atomic number. However, there are some atoms of the same type that have a different mass number. This variation is due to an imbalance of neutrons. These atoms are called **isotopes**. For isotopes, the atomic number (determined by the number of protons) is the same, but the mass number (determined by adding the protons and neutrons) is different. This is a result of there being a different number of neutrons.

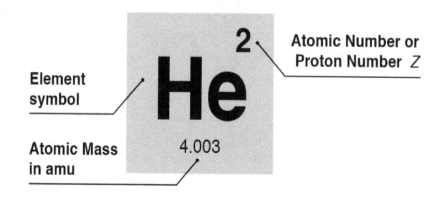

The Periodic Table arranges elements by atomic number, similar characteristics, and electron configurations in a tabular format. The vertical lines are called *columns* and are sorted by similar chemical properties/characteristics, such as appearance and reactivity. This is seen in the shiny texture of metals, the softness of post-transition metals, and the high melting points of alkali earth metals. The horizontal lines are called *rows* and are arranged by electron valance configurations. The columns are referred to as *groups,* and the rows are *periods.*

The Nature of Electricity

Electrostatics is the study of electric charges at rest. A balanced atom has a neutral charge from its number of electrons and protons. If the charge from its electrons is greater than or less than the charge of its protons, the atom has a charge. If the atom has a greater charge from the number of electrons than protons, it has a negative charge. If the atom has a lesser charge from the number of electrons than protons, it has a positive charge. Opposite charges attract each other, while like charges repel each other, so a negative attracts a positive, and a negative repels a negative. Similarly, a positive charge repels a positive charge. Just as energy cannot be created or destroyed, neither can charge; charge can only be transferred. The transfer of charge can occur through touch, or the transfer of electrons. Once electrons have transferred from one object to another, the charge has been transferred.

For example, if a person wears socks and scuffs their feet across a carpeted floor, the person is transferring electrons to the carpeting through the friction from their feet. Additionally, if that person then touches a light switch, they he or she receive a small shock. This "shock" is the person feeling the electrons transferring from the switch to their hand. Since the person lost electrons to the carpet, that person now has fewer negative charges, resulting in a net positive charge. Therefore, the electrons from the light switch are attracted to the person for the transfer. The shock felt is the electrons moving from the switch to the person's finger.

Another method of charging an object is through induction. *Induction* occurs when a charged object is brought near two touching stationary objects. The electrons in the objects will attract and cluster near another positively-charged object and repel away from a negatively-charged object held nearby. The stationary objects will redistribute their electrons to allow the charges to reposition themselves closer or farther away. This redistribution will cause one of the touching stationary objects to be negatively charged and the other to be positively charged. The overall charges contained in the stationary objects remain the same but are repositioned between the two objects.

Another way to charge an object is through *polarization*. Polarization can occur simply by the reconfiguration of the electrons within a single object.

For example, if a girl at a birthday party rubs a balloon on her hair, the balloon could then cling to a wall if it were brought close enough. This would be because rubbing the balloon causes it to become negatively charged. When the balloon is held against a neutrally-charged wall, the negatively charged balloon repels all the wall's electrons, causing a positively-charged surface on the wall. This type of charge is temporary, due to the massive size of the wall, and the charges will quickly redistribute.

An electric current is produced when electrons carry charge across a length. To make electrons move so they can carry this charge, a change in voltage must be present. On a small scale, this is demonstrated through the electrons traveling from the light switch to a person's finger in the example where the person had run their socks on a carpet. The difference between the charge in the switch and the charge in the finger causes the electrons to move. On a larger and more sustained scale, this movement would need to be more controlled. This can be achieved through batteries/cells and generators. Batteries or cells have a chemical reaction that takes place inside, causing energy to be released and charges to move freely. Generators convert mechanical energy into electric energy for use after the reaction.

For example, if a wire runs touching the end of a battery to the end of a lightbulb, and then another wire runs touching the base of the lightbulb to the opposite end of the original battery, the lightbulb will light up. This is due to a complete circuit being formed with the battery and the electrons being carried across the voltage drop (the two ends of the battery). The appearance of the light from the bulb is the visible presence of the electrons in the filament of the bulb.

Electric energy can be derived from a number of sources, including coal, wind, sun, and nuclear reactions. Electricity has numerous applications, including being transferable into light, sound, heat, or magnetic forces.

Magnetism and Electricity

Magnetic forces occur naturally in specific types of materials and can be imparted to other types of materials. If two straight iron rods are observed, they will naturally have a negative end (pole) and a positive end (pole). These charged poles follow the rules of any charged item: Opposite charges attract, and like charges repel. When set up positive to negative, they will attract each other, but if one rod is turned around, the two rods will repel each other due to the alignment of negative to negative poles and positive to positive poles. When poles are identified, magnetic fields are observed between them. If small iron filings (a material with natural magnetic properties) are sprinkled over a sheet of paper resting on top of a bar magnet, the field lines from the poles can be seen in the alignment of the iron filings, as pictured below:

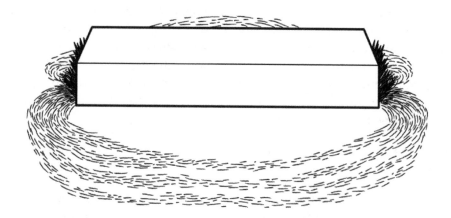

These fields naturally occur in materials with magnetic properties. There is a distinct pole at each end of such a material. If materials are not shaped with definitive ends, the fields will still be observed through the alignment of poles in the material.

For example, a circular magnet does not have ends but still has a magnetic field associated with its shape, as pictured below:

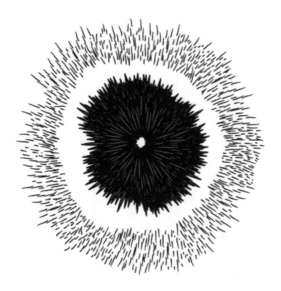

Magnetic forces can also be generated and amplified by using an electric current. For example, if an electric current is sent through a length of wire, it creates an electromagnetic field around the wire from the charge of the current. This force is from the moving of negatively-charged electrons from one end of the wire to the other. This is maintained as long as the flow of electricity is sustained. The magnetic field can also be used to attract and repel other items with magnetic properties. A smaller or larger magnetic force can be generated around this wire, depending on the strength of the current in the wire. As soon as the current is stopped, the magnetic force also stops.

Magnetic energy can be harnessed, or manipulated, from natural sources or from a generated source (a wire carrying electric current). When a core with magnetic properties (such as iron) has a wire wrapped around it in circular coils, it can be used to create a strong, non-permanent electromagnet. If current is run through the wrapped wire, it generates a magnetic field by polarizing the ends of the metal core, as described above, by moving the negative charge from one end to the other. If the direction of the current is reversed, so is the direction of the magnetic field due to the poles of the core being reversed. The term *non-permanent* refers to the fact that the magnetic field is generated only when the current is present, but not when the current is stopped.

The following is a picture of a small electromagnet made from an iron nail, a wire, and a battery:

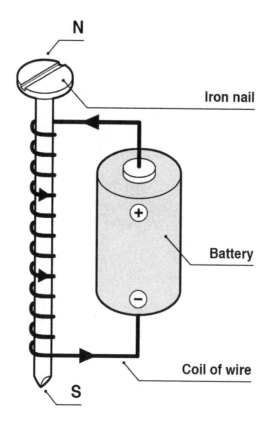

This type of **electromagnetic field** can be generated on a larger scale using more sizable components. This type of device is useful in the way it can be controlled. Rather than having to attempt to block a permanent magnetic field, the current to the system can simply be stopped, thus stopping the magnetic field. This provides the basis for many computer-related instruments and magnetic resonance imaging (MRI) technology. Magnetic forces are used in many modern applications, including the creation of super-speed transportation. Super magnets are used in rail systems and supply a cleaner form of energy than coal or gasoline. Another example of the use of super-magnets is seen in medical equipment, specifically MRI. These machines are highly sophisticated and useful in imaging the internal workings of the human body. For super-magnets to be useful, they often must be cooled down to extremely low temperatures to dissipate the amount of heat generated from their extended usage. This can be done by flooding the magnet with a super-cooled gas such as helium or liquid nitrogen. Much research is continuously done in this field to find new ceramic–metallic hybrid materials that have structures that can maintain their charge and temperature within specific guidelines for extended use.

HESI Physics Practice Questions

1. For what entity does kinematics provide a guideline?
   a. Motion
   b. Time
   c. Mass
   d. Position

2. Which answer choice describes Newton's law of inertia?
   a. For every action, there is an equal and opposite reaction.
   b. Velocity is equal to a change in position divided by the change in time.
   c. The force acting upon an object is equal to the object's mass multiplied by its acceleration.
   d. An object at rest tends to stay at rest and an object in motion tends to stay in motion unless an outside force acts upon it.

3. If a vehicle increases speed from 20 m/s to 40 m/s over a time period of 20 seconds, what is the vehicle's rate of acceleration?
   a. 2 m/s^2
   b. 1 m/s^2
   c. 10 m/s^2
   d. 20 m/s^2

4. Under which situation does an object have a negative acceleration?
   a. It is increasing velocity in a positive direction.
   b. It is at a complete stop.
   c. It is increasing velocity in a negative direction.
   d. It is moving at a constant velocity.

5. If an object is thrown into the air, at which of the following angles will it travel the SHORTEST distance horizontally?
   a. 60 degrees
   b. 75 degrees
   c. 30 degrees
   d. 45 degrees

6. What is friction?
   a. It is the normal force of an object that is perpendicular to the surface.
   b. It is the force required to maintain the movement of an object.
   c. It is the force that opposes motion.
   d. It is the velocity of an object.

7. What is the coefficient of static friction if you needed a 10 N force to push a 5 kg box from rest across a flat floor?
   a. 0.2
   b. 0.5
   c. 1.0
   d. 2.0

8. What shape of path is an object moving in that is experiencing angular momentum?
   a. Square
   b. Straight line
   c. Zig-zag pattern
   d. Circle

9. Where should a person sit on a merry-go-round to experience the greatest linear speed of the ride?
   a. Halfway between the axis and the outer most horse
   b. $\frac{1}{3}$ of the way between the axis and the outer most horse
   c. On the outermost horse
   d. On the innermost horse

10. What torque would result from a 35 N force that was applied to a lever 10 meters away from the axis of rotation?
   a. 35 N×m
   b. 350 N×m
   c. 10 N×m
   d. 3.5 N×m

11. When clothes are being spun in a washing machine, what type of force causes the water to be expelled through the small holes in the barrel of the washer?
   a. Centripetal
   b. Friction
   c. Angular momentum
   d. Centrifugal

12. What type of energy does a roller coaster car sitting still on the track at the top of a hill have?
   a. All kinetic energy, no potential energy
   b. No kinetic energy, all potential energy
   c. Half kinetic energy, half potential energy
   d. No energy at all

13. If a truck with a mass of 1000 kg and a car with a mass of 500 kg are traveling down the same street at the same velocity, which one will have greater momentum?
   a. The truck
   b. They have the same momentum.
   c. It cannot be determined without knowing their rate of acceleration.
   d. The car

14. In addition to the mass of the two objects, what other factor can change the attractive force between two objects?
   a. The height of the objects
   b. The velocity of the objects
   c. The general gravitational constant
   d. The distance between the two objects

15. Which concept explains the rising of tides in the ocean?
    a. The sun pulling the ocean water up.
    b. The Earth pushing its oceans towards the moon.
    c. The moon's gravitational effect pulling on the Earth.
    d. The sun pushing the ocean waters up.

16. In which direction does a longitudinal wave travel?
    a. Parallel to the direction of the wave's travel
    b. Perpendicular to the direction of the wave's travel
    c. At a 45-degree angle to the direction of the wave's travel
    d. At a 30-degree angle to the direction of the wave's travel

17. In which way does the Doppler effect NOT affect how an observer experiences light or sound waves?
    a. The wave appears shorter.
    b. The wave appears longer.
    c. The pitch of the sound appears higher.
    d. A longitudinal wave appears to be a transverse wave.

18. What type of light is harmful to human skin?
    a. Ultraviolet (UV) light
    b. The whole visible spectrum
    c. Radio waves
    d. Blue light

19. Which principle of light occurs when a wave travels through a slit or around an obstacle?
    a. Refraction
    b. Diffraction
    c. Reflection
    d. Greenhouse effect

20. What happens when white light is dispersed through a prism?
    a. It interacts with another light wave.
    b. It is completely absorbed.
    c. The white light is split into each of its separate rainbow-colored components.
    d. Light is reflected completely within the prism and cannot escape.

21. A microscope is particularly useful to visualize which of the following?
    a. Objects that are too big to see as a whole.
    b. Objects that are reflected in a mirror.
    c. Objects that are too far away to be seen with the human eye.
    d. Objects that are too small to see with the human eye.

22. According to the Bohr model, where do the electrons of an atom reside?
    a. In orbitals surrounding the nucleus
    b. In the nucleus with protons
    c. In the nucleus with neutrons
    d. Outside the atom

23. In the Periodic Table, what similarity do the elements in columns have with each other?
    a. Have the same atomic number
    b. Similar chemical properties
    c. Similar electron valence configurations
    d. Start with the same first letter

24. Which is NOT an example of how to charge an object?
    a. Transferring electrons
    b. Induction
    c. Polarization
    d. Refraction

25. Which two magnetic poles would attract each other?
    a. Two positive poles
    b. Two negative poles
    c. One positive pole and one negative pole
    d. Two circular positive magnets

For questions 26–28:

Object Moving with Constant Speed		Object Moving with Changing Speed	
Time (s)	Position (m)	Time (s)	Position (m)
0	0	0	0
1	8	1	2
2	16	2	6
3	24	3	12
4	32	4	20

26. If the velocity (speed in a direction) for an object is the measurement of the change in position divided by the change in time, modeled by the equation $v = \frac{\Delta x}{\Delta t}$, what is the velocity between 3s and 4s for the object moving with a constant speed?
    a. 0 m/s
    b. 4 m/s
    c. 6 m/s
    d. 8 m/s

27. What is the average velocity for the chart of the object moving with changing speed between 1 and 3 seconds?
    a. 1 m/s
    b. 3 m/s
    c. 5 m/s
    d. 7 m/s

226

28. What would be the rate at which the velocity is changing in the left-hand chart display?
    a. Average velocity
    b. Average speed
    c. Force
    d. Acceleration

For questions 29 – 30:

When the materials of surfaces move across one another they have a specific coefficient of friction that impedes their movement. In order to begin the sliding motion of these surfaces, a coefficient of static friction must be overcome. Once the materials begin moving across each other, the coefficient of kinetic friction is less than that of what it took to begin the sliding motion. The coefficient of friction does not have units, as it represents a proportion.

The table below lists the coefficients of static and kinetic friction of rubber on various materials:

Material 1	Material 2	Kinetic friction	Static friction
Rubber	Concrete	0.67	0.89
Rubber	Asphalt	0.66	0.84
Rubber	Cardboard	0.54	0.79
Rubber	Ice	0.14	

The graph below shows the relationship between the coefficient of friction and the distance moved for rubber on three of the materials:

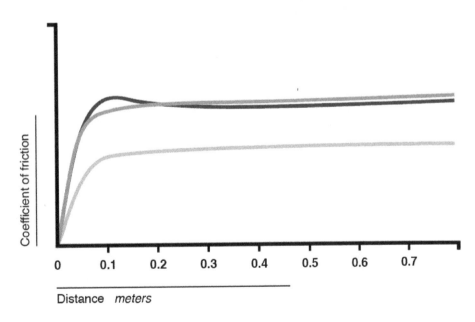

29. If material X is slightly rougher than cardboard, but smoother than asphalt, which of the following could be an approximation for the coefficient of kinetic friction of rubber on material X?
    a. 0.54
    b. 0.60
    c. 0.66
    d. Cannot be determined

30. Why do the lines in the graph all seem to level off just before a certain reading on the coefficient of friction?

  a. There are miscalculations that have altered the data
  b. They are all nearly the same material
  c. The sliding friction is overcome at that point
  d. A lubricant is added at that point

Answer Explanations

1. A: Kinematics provides a guideline for describing motion. The equations describe the change in an object's position, Choice *D*, as a function of time, Choice *B*. Mass, Choice *C*, does not play a role in kinematics.

2. D: Inertia is the idea of doing nothing and remaining unchanged. Newton's law of inertia describes what happens to an object when it stands alone, without outside forces causing changes in its motion. Choice *A* describes Newton's third law and involves action of an object. Choice *B* describes kinematics and motion. Choice *C* describes Newton's second law and involves a force acting on an object.

3. B: The equation for calculating acceleration is:

$$a = \frac{\Delta v}{\Delta t} = \frac{v_f - v_i}{\Delta t}$$

In this case, V_f = 40 m/s, V_i = 20 m/s, and Δt = 20 s. Plugging in the numbers gives an acceleration rate of 1 m/s², Choice *B*.

4. C: If an object is moving in a negative direction, it has a negative velocity. If the velocity is increasing in that negative direction, it is becoming increasingly more negative and would therefore have a negative acceleration. In Choice *A*, the object would have a positive acceleration. Acceleration is zero in both Choices *B* and *D* because the velocity of the object is not changing.

5. B: Objects thrown at the greatest angle between 0 and 90 degrees will travel the shortest distance horizontally. As the angle increases towards 90 degrees, the y-component, or height, of the motion increases proportionally and at angles greater than 45 degrees, the y-component is larger than the *x*-component, or length, of the motion. When the y-component is greater than the *x*-component, the object will travel higher vertically than it will horizontally. At 60 degrees, Choice *A*, the object will not travel as high vertically but will travel farther horizontally. At 30 degrees, Choice *C*, the object will not travel as high vertically but will travel farther horizontally. At 45 degrees, Choice *D*, the object will not travel as far vertically but will travel the farthest distance horizontally.

6. C: Friction is the force of an object that opposes motion when it interacts with another surface. Every surface has some amount of friction that resists motion. All objects have a perpendicular force that they exert on surfaces they touch, Choice *A*, but this is not defined as friction; it is called normal force. Friction specifically involves the resisting force when trying to move an object and does not involve the velocity of an object; therefore, Choices *B* and *D* are incorrect.

7. A: The equation for the coefficient of static friction is:

$$\mu_s = \frac{F_s}{F_N}$$

F_s is the friction force, which is the 10 N force that is required to push the box. The equation for F_N is:

$$F_N = mass \times gravity$$

The force of gravity is always equal to 9.8 m/s². The mass of the object is 5 kg.

Therefore:

$$\mu_s = 10 \text{ N}/(5 \text{ kg} \times 9.8 \text{ m/s}^2) = 0.2$$

8. D: Momentum is the measure of an object's mass and velocity in a specific direction. Angular momentum is the momentum of an object moving on a circular path. Since a circular path is constant, without an end, the angular momentum of a system is also constant. A straight-line path would have regular momentum, Choice *B*. Angular momentum does not refer to the angles involved in squares or a zig-zag pattern, making Choices *A* and *C* incorrect.

9. C: The rotational speed of all objects moving around an axis is the same. However, the linear speed of the object farthest away from the axis will be the greatest because they have a larger distance to cover in the same amount of time, compared with an object that is closest to the axis. On a merry-go-round, the innermost horse has the least distance to cover in a full rotation of the axis, so it will have the smallest linear speed; therefore, Choice *D* is incorrect. Horses anywhere in between the innermost and outermost horses will have linear speeds greater than that of the innermost horse but smaller than that of the outermost horse. Thus, Choices *A* and *B* are incorrect.

10. B: The equation to determine torque is:

$$Torque = F_\perp \times distance\ of\ lever\ arm\ from\ the\ axis\ of\ rotation$$

where $F_\perp$ is the perpendicular force that is being applied to the object. Thus:

$$Torque = 35 \text{ N} \times 10 \text{ m} = 350 \text{ N}\times\text{m}$$

11. D: When an object is moving in a circular motion, the force that pushes outward, away from the axis, is called the centrifugal force. It is this outward force that would expel water through the holes in the barrel from the clothes that are pushed up to the sides of the barrel. The centripetal force, Choice *A*, is the force that is pulling the clothes towards the axis. Friction, Choice *B*, does not affect the water being pulled through the holes. Angular momentum, Choice *C*, is a circular force but is not responsible for pulling the water outwards.

12. B: Potential energy is stored energy. Kinetic energy is the energy of motion. Since the roller coaster car is sitting still and not moving, it does not have any kinetic energy and just has potential energy. Once it starts moving down the hill, its energy would be converted and some of the potential energy would become kinetic energy; therefore, Choice *C* is incorrect. At the bottom of the hill, when the car was moving the fastest it possibly could, all of the energy would be kinetic energy, without any potential energy left, so Choice *A* is incorrect.

13. A: The truck will have greater momentum because it has a greater mass than the car. The equation for calculating momentum is:

$$p = m \times v$$

where m is the mass of the object and v is the velocity. If the velocity is the same for both objects, then the momentum, p, will be greater for the object with a greater mass. Acceleration, Choice *C*, does not factor into the momentum of the objects.

14. D: The amount of attractive force between two objects is calculated by the following equation:

$$F = G \frac{m_1 m_2}{r^2}$$

As the two objects grow farther apart from each other, the denominator of the equation—the square of the distance between them—increases, and the force of attraction decreases. If the distance decreases, the force of attraction increases. The height of the object and the velocity of the objects, Choices *A* and *B*, are not factored into the equation. The general gravitational constant does not change, so it does not impact any changes in the attractive force between two objects, therefore, Choice *C* is incorrect.

15. C: The moon has a gravitational pull on the Earth as it orbits around it. The pull causes the tides in oceans to rise, and the point where the moon is closest to the Earth is when high tide occurs. The Earth orbits around the sun but does not affect the tides of the ocean; therefore, Choices *A* and *D* are incorrect. The tides are caused by the moon's pull on the ocean and not the other way around, so Choice *B* is incorrect.

16. A: Longitudinal waves travel in a direction that is parallel to the wave's travel. When a spring is compressed and then released, its energy is released across the length of the spring until is completely dissipated. Transverse waves have a motion that is perpendicular to the wave's direction of travel, so Choice *B* is wrong. Longitudinal waves do not travel at 45- or 30-degree angles to the direction of the wave's travel, making Choices *C* and *D* incorrect.

17. D: The Doppler effect changes the way an observer experiences light and sound waves based on their relative position to the source of the wave. Although it appears that the wave has changed, it actually remains the same. The waves can appear shorter or longer and sound waves can appear to have higher or lower pitches; therefore, Choices *A*, *B*, and *C* are incorrect. The wave cannot change from having an appearance of being longitudinal to being transverse.

18. A: Beyond the visible spectrum of light are shorter wavelengths of light that can be harmful to humans. The sun has a small percentage of UV light, and when that crosses into the Earth's atmosphere, it can be harmful to human skin and cause burns. The whole visible spectrum, Choice *B*, including blue light, Choice *D*, is not harmful to human skin. Radio waves have long waves, and although they are not visible to the human eye, they are not harmful to the skin; therefore, Choice *C* is incorrect.

19. B: Diffraction occurs when a wave travels through a slit or around an obstacle. The light bends and then causes a spread on the other side of the opening or obstacle. Refraction, Choice *A*, occurs when a wave travels from one medium to another, and it bends as it moves through the different densities. Reflection, Choice *C*, occurs when a wave hits a medium that it cannot pass through and is bounced back. The greenhouse effect, Choice *D*, occurs when light from the sun cannot escape the Earth's atmosphere and bounces back and forth by reflection.

20. C: The dispersion of light occurs when the single white light wave is refracted and split into each of its separate colored components. These individual color waves are seen in the prism. When a light wave interacts with another wave it is called interference, Choice *A*. The prism does not absorb the light completely, so Choice *B* is incorrect. When a wave enters an object and is completely reflected within it without being able to escape, it is called total internal reflection; therefore, Choice *D* is incorrect.

21. D: Microscopes magnify objects that are too small to see with the human eye. Microscopes do not reduce the size of objects that are too big. Objects that are reflected in a mirror can be seen with the unaided eye. Telescopes allow you to see objects that are far away. Therefore, Choice *A*, *B*, and *C* are incorrect.

22. A: Electrons reside in orbitals outside the nucleus. They are negatively charged and are attracted to the protons that reside in the nucleus. The protons and neutrons carry most of the mass of the atoms (at least 99% of the total mass). The nucleus contains only protons and neutrons, not electrons, so Choices *B* and *C* are incorrect. The orbitals that the electrons reside in are within the boundaries of the atom and not outside; thus, Choice *D* is incorrect.

23. B: The elements are arranged such that the elements in columns have similar chemical properties, such as appearance and reactivity. Each element has a unique atomic number, not the same one, so Choice *A* is incorrect. Elements are arranged in rows, not columns, with similar electron valence configurations, so Choice *C* is incorrect. The names of the elements are not arranged alphabetically in columns, Choice *D*.

24. D: Refraction involves the bending of light through different mediums and does not affect the charge of an object. Electrons can be transferred from one object to another, giving an object a negative charge, so Choice *A* is incorrect. Induction, Choice *B*, involves the redistribution of charge by bringing a charged object close to two stationary objects. If the charged object is negatively charged, the electrons of the stationary objects will be repelled away and one of the stationary objects will take on a positive charge while the other one will become negatively charged. Polarization, Choice *C*, occurs when electrons in an object are reconfigured temporarily.

25. C: Magnets follow the same rules of charge as other items. Positive and negative poles attract each other. Two poles with the same charge, positive or negative, would repel each other; therefore, Choices *A* and *B* are incorrect. Although circular magnets do not have ends, they still have poles and follow the same rules of charge. So, circular positive magnets would repel each other, making Choice *D* incorrect.

26. D: In order to calculate the velocity, the following equation should be utilized:

$$v = \frac{\Delta x}{\Delta t} = \frac{x_2 - x_1}{t_2 - t_1} = \frac{32m - 24m}{4s - 3s} = \frac{8m}{1s} = 8\ m/s$$

27. C: In order to calculate this, the same equation in question 21 can be used, but the values used will be pulled from the right half of the chart:

$$v = \frac{\Delta x}{\Delta t} = \frac{x_2 - x_1}{t_2 - t_1} = \frac{12m - 2m}{3s - 1s} = \frac{10m}{2s} = 5\ m/s$$

28. D: The change in velocity over the change in time would display the acceleration, which is modeled by the equation $a = \frac{\Delta v}{\Delta t}$. Choice *A* is calculated through finding the average of all of the velocity values, Choice *B* involves calculating the magnitude of the average without the direction, and Choice *C* cannot be calculated with the information provided.

29. B: Choice *B* gives a value that is partway between the coefficient of kinetic friction of cardboard and the coefficient of kinetic friction of asphalt, which would be a reasonable approximation for material X. Choice *A* would be too low, representing the coefficient of kinetic friction of cardboard, and Choice *C* is too high for the coefficient of kinetic friction of asphalt. Choice *D* is not correct, because a relationship can be established between the materials.

30. C: The value of static friction for surfaces in contact must be overcome in order to start motion. After this coefficient of static friction is overcome, the materials begin moving across each other, and the coefficient of kinetic friction is less than that of what it took to begin the sliding motion. As two out of the three graphed lines are similar in value as to where the coefficient of static friction is overcome, it shows that the surfaces move more easily across each other with the lower coefficient of kinetic friction.

Greetings!

First, we would like to give a huge "thank you" for choosing us and this study guide for your HESI A2 exam. We hope that it will lead you to success on this exam and for your years to come.

Our team has tried to make your preparations as thorough as possible by covering all of the topics you should be expected to know. In addition, our writers attempted to create practice questions identical to what you will see on the day of your actual test. We have also included many test-taking strategies to help you learn the material, maintain the knowledge, and take the test with confidence.

We strive for excellence in our products, and if you have any comments or concerns over the quality of something in this study guide, please send us an email so that we may improve.

As you continue forward in life, we would like to remain alongside you with other books and study guides in our library. We are continually producing and updating study guides in several different subjects. If you are looking for something in particular, all of our products are available on Amazon. You may also send us an email!

Sincerely,
APEX Test Prep
info@apexprep.com

FREE

Free Study Tips DVD

In addition to the tips and content in this guide, we have created a FREE DVD with helpful study tips to further assist your exam preparation. **This FREE Study Tips DVD provides you with top-notch tips to conquer your exam and reach your goals.**

Our simple request in exchange for the strategy-packed DVD is that you email us your feedback about our study guide. We would love to hear what you thought about the guide, and we welcome any and all feedback—positive, negative, or neutral. It is our #1 goal to provide you with top quality products and customer service.

To receive your **FREE Study Tips DVD**, email freedvd@apexprep.com. Please put "FREE DVD" in the subject line and put the following in the email:

    a. The name of the study guide you purchased.

    b. Your rating of the study guide on a scale of 1-5, with 5 being the highest score.

    c. Any thoughts or feedback about your study guide.

    d. Your first and last name and your mailing address, so we know where to send your free DVD!

Thank you!

CPSIA information can be obtained
at www.ICGtesting.com
Printed in the USA
BVHW061833140722
642166BV00012B/1018